Lemon Cures

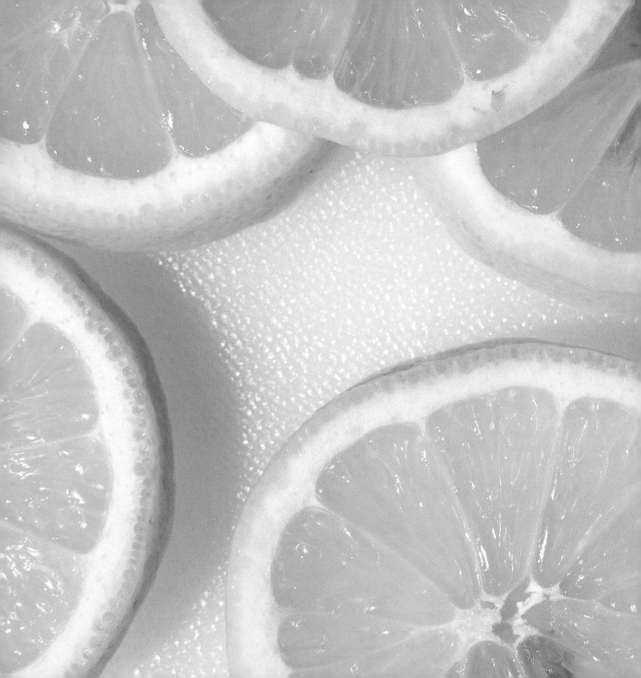

Lemon
Cures

Werner Meidinger

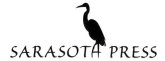

SARASOTA PRESS

U.S. and Canadian Cataloging-in-Publication Data available upon request.

ISBN: 1-55356-000-0

Published in the United States in 2001 by
Sarasota Press
an imprint of Key Porter Books Limited
4808 South Tamiami Trail
PMB #205
Sarasota, Florida
34231-4352

Published in Canada in 2001 by
Key Porter Books Limited
70 The Esplanade
Toronto, Ontario
Canada M5E 1R4

Originally published in German in 1998 by W. Ludwig Buchverlag GmbH for Verlaghaus Goethestrasse GmbH & Co. KG, Munich

www.keyporter.com

Translation: Elizabeth Schweiger
Design: Patricia Cavazzini
Electronic formatting: Jean Peters
Photography: Mir Lada
Food and Prop Styling: Patricia Cavazzini

Printed and bound in Canada

01 02 03 04 05 6 5 4 3 2

Contents

The Yellow Power Pack

The lemon is a fruit that has been used by mankind for a very long time. Its history reaches back more than four thousand years. Paleobotanists have discovered traces of its existence in Southeast Asia and in northwestern India, near the Himalayas. But lemon trees also grew in the fertile valleys of the Euphrates and the Tigris. Drawings discovered by archaeologists in the tombs in the Valley of the Kings indicate that lemons and lemon juice were used for mummification in ancient Egypt.

An Ancient Tradition as a Healing Plant

Ancient Egyptians used lemons for many different aspects of healing, for example as a tonic for colic or fever, and also as an aphrodisiac. Many believed that eating lemons and drinking lemon juice was an effective protection against a variety of poisons—and even today this belief is maintained in remote areas of eastern Turkey, the Middle East and southwestern Asia. Recent research has confirmed many of these ancient beliefs.

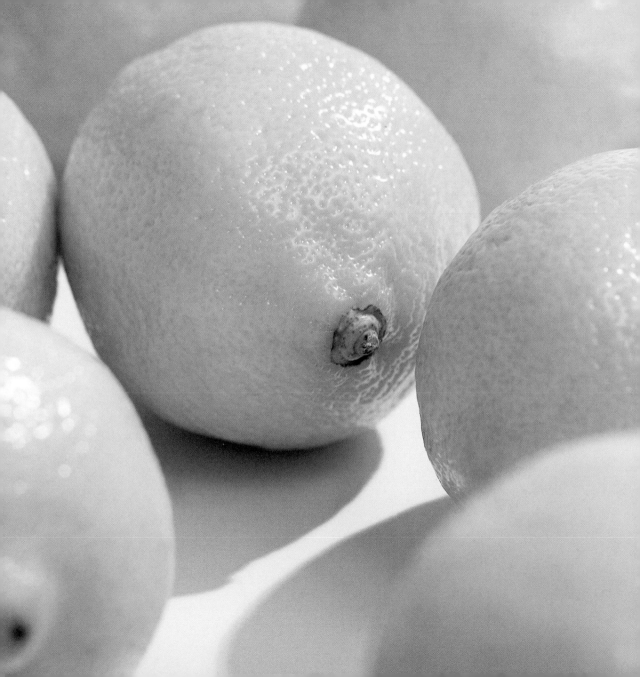

In the baroque period, lemon and orange trees were highly fashionable. They adorned the scrupulously symmetrical gardens of kings and emperors. Magnificent buildings, called orangeries, were erected to protect the valuable plants in winter.

Lemons in Greek Antiquity

It is probable that the ancient Greeks were introduced to lemons by Alexander the Great, the king of Macedonia, who would have brought them back from his victorious military campaigns against the Persians. At any rate, to the Greeks lemons were known as Persian apples. They planted lemon trees along the edges of their olive groves, believing that the citrus would keep pests at bay. The juice was used to preserve food, as a disinfectant, as a cleansing agent in water for laundry and scrubbing, and for treating various common ailments and illnesses.

Lemons in the Roman Empire

The Greeks brought lemons to Rome, where they were at first used exclusively to keep moths out of wool clothing. After some time the Romans learned from Persian slaves that lemons could be used to prepare tasty meals and refreshing drinks. The fruit became such a favorite that it featured as a staple in their field kitchens, and thus it was brought to Spain, France, northern Italy and even North Africa during the course of the many Roman military campaigns.

From "Fruit of Evil" to Healing Plant

Although lemons have generally been popular for treating ailments and adding flavor to meals, there was a brief period in the Middle Ages when they were considered a fruit of evil. Superstition attributed all kinds of noxious and even toxic qualities to them. These superstitions did not persist, however, and lemons soon became known around the world through Spanish and Portuguese seafarers. Christopher Columbus planted the first lemon trees on Haiti in 1493 and they spread with lightning speed across all the Caribbean islands. In 1579 the first lemon trees of the New World were discovered in St. Augustine, Florida. The plants thrived and spread until a severe frost destroyed the entire stock in 1894. Fortunately, some twenty years earlier, hardier types had been introduced to California, whence they spread across the entire western United States.

Today, we can no longer imagine our kitchens, cosmetics and especially natural health care without lemons. In this volume we have gathered many tips and ideas on the uses of this tart fruit: tasty meals and refreshing drinks, soothing creams and fragrant baths, healing teas and vitamin-rich juices. In addition, you will learn about the many advantages this small fruit has to offer and how its ingredients affect the human body. So, use the natural power that lies hidden in the lemon!

CHAPTER 1

How to Buy
and Use Lemons

Advice on Shopping

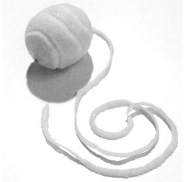

The size of the fruit does not indicate the amount of juice it will yield. Small lemons with a thin peel contain more juice than varieties with thick peels and comparatively little flesh.

Them major suppliers of lemons today are the western United States, Spain, Italy and Greece. With a total of 3.5 tons of lemons per year, these regions deliver over half of the world's harvest. Lemons can be purchased year-round at well under a dollar each, depending upon the season. To derive the greatest benefit from the healthy ingredients, here are some tips on what to look for when you buy lemons.

What the peel tells us
• Ripe lemons are not hard; the skin is an even light yellow and shiny. If the skin looks matte or has green spots, the fruit is not fully ripened.
• When the skin is a more saturated, deep yellow, or even a brownish yellow, and if the fruit is very soft to the touch, then it is overripe. The same applies if the skin displays any hardened areas, and if it is wrinkled or torn. A simple rule of thumb: the paler the yellow, the tarter the fruit. If you prefer a less sour lemon taste, you should select lemons with a deep yellow skin.

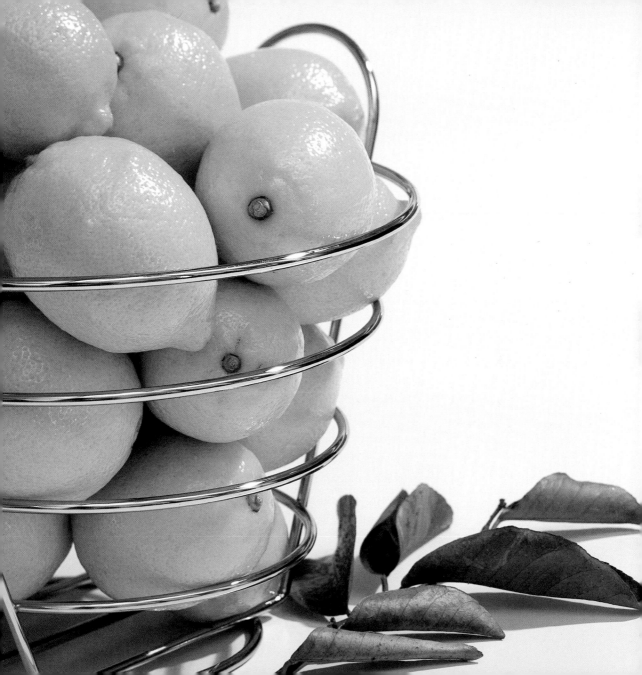

If you frequently use lemons in your special dishes and want to have them on hand, you can store them for as long as a year in the freezer.

• Since lemons are often heavily sprayed with chemicals to protect them against pests, it is worthwhile to shop around for organic fruit; the best is available in health food stores. To be on the safe side you can soak the whole fruit in lukewarm water, adding a small amount of dishwashing liquid. After scrubbing, they should be carefully rinsed in cold, clear water.

Storage

When you cut a lemon in half and want to keep one of the halves for later use, the citric acid at the cut is normally not enough to prevent spoilage for long. If you brush the cut with vinegar, its acetic acid helps to keep the half-lemon fresh for days.

• At room temperature, lemons will keep for eight to ten days without any loss of quality. Should you wish to keep them longer, it is best to refrigerate them. However, they should not be jammed together into a small compartment. The best container is one that allows air to circulate around the fruit on all sides, for example a wire bowl or woven basket. Stored in this manner, the fruit will easily keep for a month.

• Lemons can also be frozen—for up to a year. To freeze the juice, pour it into ice-cube trays. You will then have perfect portions of frozen lemon juice. When thawed, the taste is as if it were freshly squeezed. Lemon slices or wedges can also be frozen, the peeled pieces being cut into appropriate sizes and frozen in vacuum-sealed plastic freezer bags. When thawed, however, such pieces of lemon are no longer ideal for direct consumption, because the flesh of the fruit is spongy. They should be used only for cooking. Whole and unpeeled lemons can be frozen, but only the juice can be used later on. After thawing, they are soft and easy to press.

Handling

Tips for pressing juice

For pressing the juice it is best to use lemons at room temperature. The juice is contained in small pockets, like tiny sacs. To extract the most juice, these small pockets should be made to burst even before pressing. To do so, place the lemon on a hard surface and roll it back and forth several times, exerting firm pressure. With conventional lemon presses, the walls of the juice pockets are simply punctured through the repeated pressure against the ridges of the lemon press. You will get more juice by placing the lemon for a few minutes into water warmed to 105 to 120 degrees Fahrenheit (40–50°C). With this treatment, an average-sized lemon should yield 2 to 3 tablespoons (30 to 45 ml) of juice.

Don't forget to use the peel

If you buy untreated or organic lemons, you can use the peel in a number of food recipes (see page 88). The skin should therefore be prepared for storage. Before extracting the juice, the skin should be peeled off with a standard vegetable peeler. Take care not to cut too deeply, avoiding the white, subcutaneous part of the skin. This inner layer has an extremely bitter taste, and even small amounts can ruin the flavor of a meal. After peeling, the skin will be in strips. These should be spread out on some wax paper and left to dry for two to three days. Then place them in a linen or cotton pouch and hang in a dry, airy place. The drying process can be accelerated in the oven. Place the strips of peel on

The candied lemon peel used for baking comes from a specific lemon variety. It bears fruit the size of a rugby ball and has a peel that can be up to 4 inches (10 cm) thick. It is commercially available in large chunks or small pieces.

If you have grated the peel, use the lemon as soon as possible: without the protective outer layer, lemons spoil quickly. You should throw out moldy lemons promptly, as the mold can be particularly harmful.

a baking sheet and dry them on the lowest heat setting for four to six hours, leaving the oven door slightly open. Before using the lemon peel, soak the pieces in water until they have softened. The skin can then be used just as if it were freshly peeled. The same procedures can be applied to grated lemon peel. It can also be dried into a powder and preserved in small jars.

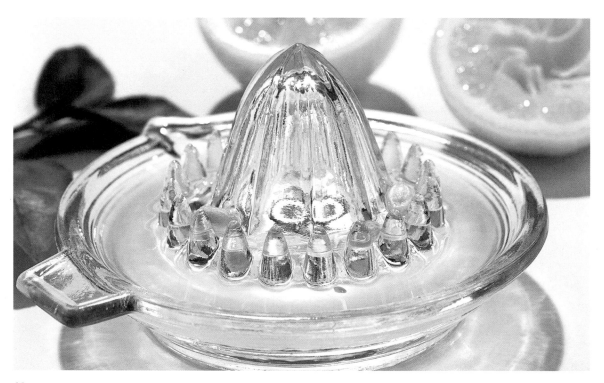

Lemon-scented plants

• *Lemon grass* Lemon grass (*Cymbopogon citratus*) is a Southeast Asian plant from the licorice family, which has a slight lemony flavor when chewed. It contains healing volatile (or essential) oils. Teas prepared with lemon grass are used to alleviate stomach pains accompanied by diarrhea, fever, loss of appetite and nervousness. Externally, the oils can soothe pain associated with lumbago, rheumatism, sprains and pulled muscles. The healing powers of lemon grass are often used in combination with those of the lemon itself.

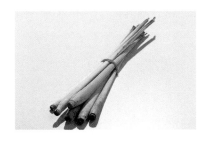

• *Lemon balm* Lemon balm, like lemon grass, has nothing to do with lemon trees. It is the name commonly used for melissa (*Melissa officinalis*). It contains essential melissa oil. Lemon balm tea is a proven tonic for calming nerves and treating insomnia. When combined with the substances in lemons known to stimulate the body's immune system, it is also soothing and healing for feverish ailments, such as colds and influenza, as well as for headaches or respiratory inflammations.

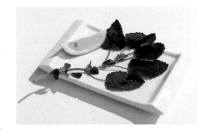

• *Lemon pelargonium* These fragrant plants are related to the geraniums we hang on balconies, with smaller flowers in pastel pinks and pleasant, aromatic leaves. They are used to add aroma to baked goods and sweets, for potpourri and fragrant pouches, and as indoor plants that are believed to neutralize the smell of cigarette smoke. Of the many fragrant pelargonium plants, *Pelargonium citronella* and the *Pelargonium* "Queen of Lemon" are the types with the strongest lemon fragrance.

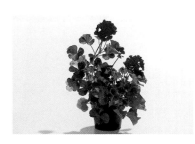

CHAPTER 2

What Lemons Contain

In home remedies, lemons have been used for a broad spectrum of ailments for many centuries. Each part of the fruit is used: the pulp, the juice, the peel and the essential oil it contains.

Take an untreated, organic lemon—perhaps from a health food store—and rub the rough side of a dry sugar cube over the peel. If you need the aroma of lemon oil as a special touch for a dish, such as a dessert, you can use the enriched sugar cube. Of course, you can also just suck on it to enjoy the taste and the beneficial qualities of the lemon oil.

Pulp and Juice

The pulp of a lemon contains many essential nutrients. These substances are also present in slightly less concentrated form in the juice. The juice will yield over 90 percent of the vitamin C contained in the entire fruit, two-thirds of the calcium and only one-third of the iron. The only way to benefit fully from the valuable nutrients is to eat the entire fruit, including the pulp. Even though it may taste very sour to begin with, our taste buds quickly adapt and after a few days most people think nothing of eating a raw lemon.

Laboratory studies of lemons
Two university studies have recently yielded surprising results on the healing powers of the lemon. These findings encourage and support the daily use of lemons.

- Scientists at the Institute for Pharmaceutics and Biochemistry at the University of Buenos Aires, Argentina, were looking for a natural disinfectant for drinking water polluted with cholera bacteria (*Vibrio cholerae*). Lemon juice turned out to be ideal. The cholera bacteria in the drinking water died as soon as fresh lemon juice was added to the polluted water to a level of 2 percent. After thirty minutes the drinking water was completely free of bacteria.

- The epidemiological service of the Ministry of Health in Guinea-Bissau in West Africa released a similar recommendation during a cholera epidemic in October 1994. Doctors recommended adding lemon juice to meals and generally using as many lemons as possible in food preparation as prevention against cholera infection.

The acidity of lemon flesh stimulates the salivary glands. Elderly people in particular often produce inadequate amounts of saliva, which plays a crucial role in digestion.

Lemon Peel and Its Essential Oil

Lemon peel has thousands of minuscule glands, which produce its essential oil (*Citri aetheroleum*). The oil is extracted by cold-pressing the peel. Some three thousand lemons are required to produce 1¾ pints (1 l) of essential lemon oil. In addition to many other substances, it contains large amounts of citral, the substance that creates the typical lemon scent and taste. Today, synthetic citralis is also available and it is therefore important when buying lemon oil to check that it is natural and without artificial additives. Lemon oil can be used for physical as well as emotional ailments. In aromatherapy the oil promotes spiritual well-being; in topical applications it destroys harmful bacteria and fungi.

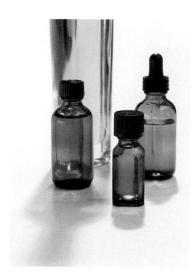

Always buy lemon oil in small quantities.
Compared with some other oils, lemon oil has a short shelf life: it spoils after about nine months. You should store it in a dark and cool place.

The characteristics of lemon oil

• Scientists at the Institute for Medical Research of the Amani Medical Research Center in Tanga, Tanzania, discovered that lemon oil is an excellent natural insect repellent. Larvae, pupae and eggs of a mosquito species were all destroyed by direct exposure to lemon oil.

• Staphylococci, which can cause skin impurities such as pimples, abscesses or sties in harmless cases, but also urinary tract infection, infectious arthritis or even heart muscle infections in serious cases, are killed off within five minutes of exposure to lemon oil.

• Even *Salmonella typhi*, the bacteria that cause typhoid fever, are destroyed after approximately one hour when treated extensively with lemon oil.

• Pneumococci, which are the cause of lung infections, meningitis, inner ear infections and peritonitis, are also destroyed after two to three hours of exposure to lemon oil.

Vitamin C

Lemons are the optimal source of vitamin C. The pulp and juice of two and a half lemons yield the average daily requirement for adults if no vitamin C is ingested from other food sources. With standard nutrition, however, it is generally sufficient to eat one raw lemon over the course of a day to obtain the daily requirement of vitamin C.

Some specifications

Vitamin C (ascorbic acid) is a water-soluble, essential vitamin. In contrast to animals, humans are unable to produce vitamin C themselves and must therefore ingest it with food. Professor Anthony Diplock of Guy's Hospital in London has evaluated over twenty studies undertaken with rigorous placebo controls in order to determine the appropriate daily dose of vitamin C. His findings resulted in a simple rule of thumb to calculate the maximum daily dose of vitamin C that an organism is able to process: 20 milligrams of vitamin C for each kilogram of body weight. (That's about 9 mg per pound.) Any vitamin C in excess of this amount is not absorbed by the organism and the body simply flushes it out.

When there is a deficiency of vitamin C, the first indicators are fatigue, difficulty in coping with stress, an impaired and delayed ability to heal, as well as an increased susceptibility to infections as a result of a weakened immune system.

It's hard to have too much of a good thing when it comes to vitamin C. While an overdose can cause skin rash and nausea with vomiting, this is rare, since excess vitamin C is normally eliminated directly in the urine and feces. The first indicator of too much vitamin C is usually diarrhea, as the body tries to rid itself of the excess vitamin as quickly as possible.

According to the most up-to-date scientific findings, an excessive dose of vitamin C does not lead to harmful side effects. Even the consumption of as much as 6 grams of vitamin C daily is not damaging to one's health.

Vitamin C and cancer

Vitamin C is one of the so-called cell-protecting vitamins, which repel free radicals and protect healthy cells from becoming cancerous. This is especially important for smokers, who inhale some 100 billion free radicals with each puff on a cigarette. In the body, free radicals immediately set off on a campaign of destruction, attacking cell walls until they find a gap through which they can

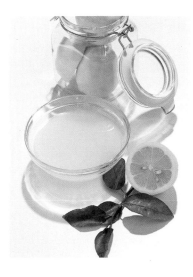

After an extensive study, scientists at the U.S. Department of Health found that only a daily intake of 200 mg of vitamin C guarantees a sufficient load for the body. Earlier recommendations, which varied in different countries between 60 and 100 mg, were clearly too low.

penetrate, harming the hereditary material and thereby triggering uncontrolled cell division.

Studies of vitamin C levels in the blood plasma of smokers revealed that they are considerably lower than in non-smokers. The cause is the more rapid consumption of vitamin C in smokers.

Vitamin C and cardiovascular disease

Cardiovascular disease beats even cancer to be the leading cause of death worldwide. In 1998, 725,000 people died in the United States of cardiovascular diseases. High levels of the harmful LDL cholesterol, mainly caused by a poor, high-fat diet, nicotine and lack of exercise, causes deposits to form in the blood vessels of the heart. These deposits increase over time, constricting the arteries until they are fully blocked—a heart attack in the making.

How vitamin C contributes to reducing cholesterol Vitamin C plays an essential part in converting cholesterol into primary bile acid in the small intestine. If too little vitamin C is present in the organism, the cholesterol cannot be excreted and begins to accumulate. This is one of the causes of high cholesterol levels. As noted in medical studies, vitamin C only contributes to lowering cholesterol levels that are abnormally elevated; when cholesterol concentrations are normal or only slightly elevated, additional vitamin C intake has no noticeable effect. Harmful side effects—perhaps even a deficiency in cholesterol as an essential substance owing to increased vitamin C intake—is therefore not a cause for concern.

Other applications of vitamin C

It is no coincidence that sailors historically stocked vast amounts of lemon juice for their journeys to prevent scurvy. In modern industrial nations we no longer need to fear that disease. Still, there are a number of other ailments for which vitamin C is useful.

- Vitamin C promotes healing. Without vitamin C, for example, open wounds would not develop scabs and heal.
- Fractures heal with the help of vitamin C because it stimulates the production of collagen. During the healing period it also promotes the constant regeneration and new formation of bone tissue, cartilage and connective tissue.
- Vitamin C helps in the development of strong and healthy teeth by stimulating the incorporation of calcium.
- Osteoporosis is reduced in women who take vitamin C regularly over a prolonged period of time.
- Vitamin C is helpful in treating stomach and digestive disorders.
- The risk of cataracts—an increased clouding of the eye's lens—can be reduced by up to 80 percent by taking vitamin C. This is explained by the ability of vitamin C to neutralize free radicals. When these aggressive particles are allowed to act for extended periods, they may damage the tissue of the ocular lens to such a degree that it clouds over.
- Vitamin C plays a major role in helping the body's immune system fight off viruses and bacteria. It promotes the production of the protein interferon, which protects cells by preventing the virus or bacteria from penetrating into the cell and multiplying there.
- According to a U.S. research study on men, regular intake of

English law dictated that every ship must have on board as much lemon juice as was required, from the tenth day of the journey until the end, to give three tablespoons daily to each person on board. This was to prevent the outbreak of scurvy.

In the past, many scientists believed that an overdose of vitamin C would lead to an overproduction of oxalic acid in the body, which in turn would lead to the formation of bladder and kidney stones. This view, says physiology professor Anthony Diplock, is no longer tenable.

vitamin C raises the average life expectancy by six years. Scientists assume that the tissue-regenerating effect of vitamin C explains this result.

Bioflavonoids

Dr. Elson Haas, medical director at the Preventive Medical Center of Marin in San Rafael, California, has conducted studies on a variety of different fruits and vegetables. He has found that citrus fruits—including lemons—in addition to tomatoes, broccoli, soy and onions, are among the ten foods containing the highest levels of bioflavonoids.

In lemons, bioflavonoids (above all, rutin, hesperidin, citrin, naringing and quercitin, from which the valuable quercetin is produced by the bacteria in the digestive tract through the segregation of sugar molecules) are present in the entire fruit, that is to say, in both the pulp and the peel, but they are most concentrated in the white layer between peel and pulp. To benefit from their healthy effects, one should therefore not remove the white skin but eat it as well—even if it does taste bitter.

Discovery by chance
More than thirty years ago, Albert Szent-Györgyi (1893–1986), the Nobel Prize winner for his discovery of vitamin C, who had immigrated to the United States from his native Hungary in 1947, came to the conclusion that there must be another substance in addition to vitamin C that has a similar effect and increases the efficiency of the vitamin. He arrived at his conclusion by a simple means: when a friend asked him for advice

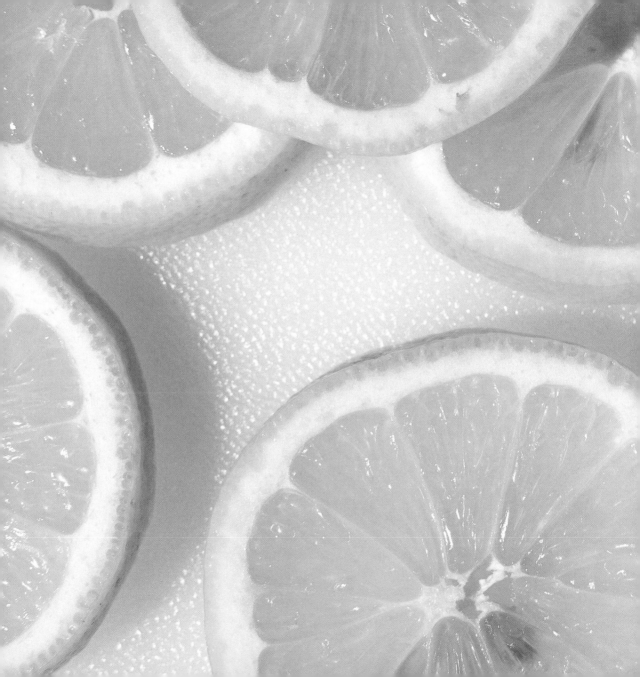

What gives oranges and lemons their characteristic color? Bioflavonoids. They fulfill important biological tasks in the human organism.

on how to stop his gums from bleeding, Szent-Györgyi gave him vitamin C extracted from the juice and pulp of a lemon for an external application. Within a short time the friend's gums stopped bleeding.

Pioneer work in the laboratory brings success

Szent-Györgyi concluded that the mixture of fruit flesh, juice and vitamin C must contain a substance that was responsible for healing the bleeding gums in the first application. He began to analyze the mixture and to isolate specific substances, which he then asked his friend to apply on the affected areas. The result: the bleeding ceased altogether. Still, Szent-Györgyi had no idea that he had isolated flavonoids; he was still thinking only of a vitamin. Since he had observed that the new substance influenced the permeability of the vascular walls, in stopping the bleeding of the gums, he called it vitamin P (permeability factor).

A new name for vitamin P

It was only much later that scientists discovered that the material in question was neither a vitamin nor even one single substance, but several substances present in many types of fruit and responsible for the yellow hue of lemon skin. Hence, these substances were named after the Latin word for "yellow" (*flavus*) as bioflavonoids.

Quercetin—the star among bioflavonoids

A substance to fend off allergies and inflammation It has been discovered that quercetin has an antibiotic and anti-allergenic effect;

it is a sort of natural antihistamine. The uncomfortable symptoms that accompany inflammation or allergies—swelling, a burning sensation, redness and itching—are caused to a large degree by an excessive discharge of the tissue hormone called histamine, which is produced in the body from the amino acid histidine.

Medication by antihistamines decreases histamine discharge and thus alleviates the related symptoms. The bioflavonoid quercetin simultaneously prevents the production and the discharge of histamine in the body, just like the synthetic medications do.

Regular consumption of lemons—including the white inner skin—reduces the symptoms of allergies and slows the excessive production of histamine in the body.

A weapon in the fight against viruses Some bioflavonoids, especially quercetin, also possess antiviral properties. This has been proven in laboratory tests on a variety of viruses. Scientific studies carried out on animals infected with a range of viral diseases all reached the same conclusion with regard to the antiviral capabilities of quercetin.

Preventing cataracts Quercetin can be an enormous help in preventing the formation of cataracts as a result of diabetes. In diabetes mellitus, cataracts are caused by an excessive production of sorbitol in a compromised sugar metabolism. Sorbitol is then present in increased concentrations throughout the entire body, including the lens of the eye. Sorbitol production is triggered by the enzyme aldosereductase.

The high sorbitol concentration in the lens leads to tissue fluid penetrating into the lens cells, simultaneously displacing important amino acids, vitamins, minerals and other nutrients from the interior of these cells to the outside. All these materials, however,

The elderly frequently suffer from cataracts. In fact, the condition is so common that it is almost regarded as a normal part of aging. Because the loss of sight happens so slowly and painlessly, the clouding of the lens often remains undiagnosed until an advanced stage.

In the past, every housewife knew about pectin: pectin gels the jam when it cools after having been cooked. That is the reason why pectin extracted from apples is added to the jelly made from raspberries or cherries, which contain very little of this substance.

contribute to the protection and regeneration of the delicate lens cells, which are thus made far more susceptible to damage by this deficit. Self-regulating repair mechanisms fail, and in the long term the delicate protein fibers of the lens become increasingly dull. Quercetin can slow down the activity of the enzyme aldosereductase, which stimulates sorbitol production, thus preventing the formation of cataracts in the first place.

Quercetin inhibits diabetes mellitus Quercetin can prevent a deterioration of diabetes by protecting the beta cells of the pancreas, in which insulin is produced, against damage from free radicals. Moreover, it stimulates the production of insulin, which is compromised in cases of diabetes mellitus.

Pectin

The lemon is among the most pectin-rich fruits. The tissue of lemon peel alone is composed of approximately 30 percent pectin. If you want to enjoy the benefit of pectin and take preventive steps against heart disease and intestinal cancers, it is best to ingest the peel as well as the rest of the lemon.

Aside from lemons, the following fruits are especially rich in pectin: apples, quince, currants, gooseberries, cranberries and grapefruit.

Ballast materials for good digestion
Pectin is a solid component in the walls of all plant cells and belongs to the large group of ballast materials vital to human digestion. The intestine, through which all food passes, is divided into two sections: the small and the large intestine. From the

stomach, food passes first into the small intestine, where the food mash is broken down into its basic substances. The individual components are absorbed by the blood and transported to all parts of the body.

Plant fibers maintain intestinal health

The large intestine follows the small intestine. Its task is to extract water from the food mash and to thicken it. In addition, the large intestine separates out the minerals and vitamins and transports them into the bloodstream. The remaining food mash is then passed on and excreted. Throughout this process the ballast materials are essential, keeping the food mash elastic, stimulating stronger movement in the muscles of the intestine and accelerating the digestive process. These plant fibers, among them pectin, cannot be digested by the body; they are excreted in nearly undigested form. And together with the ballast materials, noxious substances such as environmental toxins, metabolic "leftovers" and even pathogens are excreted.

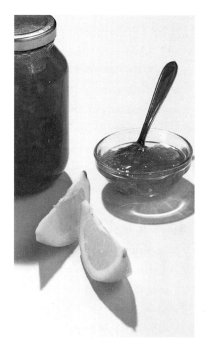

The effect in the human body

• As we eat, pectin creates a satisfying feeling of fullness. When we ingest food that is rich in pectin—for example, many recipes containing lemons—we are following an easy regime to prevent overweight, without experiencing a nagging hunger.

• Pectin supports the work of the pancreas and stimulates the production of gall liquid.

• Pectin seems to attract and hold on to environmental toxins and digestive remnants, as well as viruses and bacteria, until the digestive process is complete and they are excreted. This may be the

Citrus fruits help protect against cancer. A scientific study of dietary habits in twenty-seven countries found that stomach cancer is much rarer in countries where citrus fruit is eaten frequently. Swedish scientists have confirmed the preventive effect. They found that the occurrence of pancreatic cancer is lower by 50 to 75 percent in people who eat one citrus fruit daily as compared with those who eat less than one per week.

reason for the ability of pectin to guard against intestinal cancer, as observed in laboratory studies on animals. Scientists at the Health Science Center of the University of Texas have observed that the risk of cancer of the large intestine was reduced 50 percent in rats given a diet that was particularly high in pectin.

• Pectin, when taken regularly in the diet, protects against cardiovascular disease by keeping the harmful LDL cholesterol at low levels. This cholesterol is a primary cause of deposits forming in blood vessels, which can lead to heart attacks or strokes.

Lemon Acid

The acid content of each lemon lies somewhere around 7 percent—hence its sour taste. The acid protects the fruit from spoiling. This preserving action, however, does not last very long. In the human metabolism, lemon acid combines in a complex interaction with other acids and enzymes to ensure healthy and problem-free digestion.

Stimulates stomach juices

Lemon acid, in contrast to other acids such as the hydrochloric variety (HCL), is relatively mild, not being powerful enough to break down nutrients on its own. However, once lemon acid reaches the stomach, either in lemon flesh or as pure juice, it supports the first step of digestion in the stomach by stimulating the production of HCL, which is necessary for digestion.

Preparation for digestion

Approximately ten seconds after swallowing, food reaches the stomach through the esophagus. There are some five million tiny glands in the walls of the stomach that produce digestive enzymes and up to 2½ quarts (3 l) of HCL per day, which break down the food and prepare it for subsequent digestion in the intestine. The HCL in turn stimulates the production of the enzyme pepsin in the stomach, which is able to break down the protein components of the food.

When the glands in the stomach walls come into contact with lemon acid, they are stimulated to such a degree that the production of HCL is increased. As a consequence, pepsin production increases as well. Indirectly, lemon acid therefore supports and promotes the activity of the stomach, preparing the ground for problem-free digestion.

You benefit much more by eating whole lemons or other fruit instead of merely drinking the juice. The body is deprived of even more if you take synthetic vitamins, as they cannot replace fresh fruit.

CHAPTER 3

Prevention with the Power of Lemons

The following could be symptoms of a weakened immune system: constantly feeling unwell (for example, having recurring colds or other infections); persistent fungus infections (such as of the nails, sexual organs or inner organs); always feeling tired; quickly becoming stressed and having difficulty concentrating; needing inordinate amounts of sleep.

The human immune system is among the most fascinating—and complex—that nature has created. Antibodies stand on guard round the clock to repel certain pathogens within the body and to defend against pathogenic intruders from without. The outcome of the battle is critical, for if any of these succeed in penetrating into the human organism, they find what one could only describe as a paradise, where they are able to multiply unchecked until, in extreme cases, the body is so weakened that it dies.

Therefore, a strong immune system is essential for good overall health. Lemons help to stimulate the body's immune forces and to prevent illness—in the most natural way possible.

The Body's Daily Struggle

Pathogens are everywhere, invisibly surrounding each one of us. They float in the air, enter our bodies as we breathe, or intrude via the mucous membrane in the nostrils or lungs. They lurk on objects and clothing, whence they can penetrate into the body through open wounds, no matter how tiny. They are

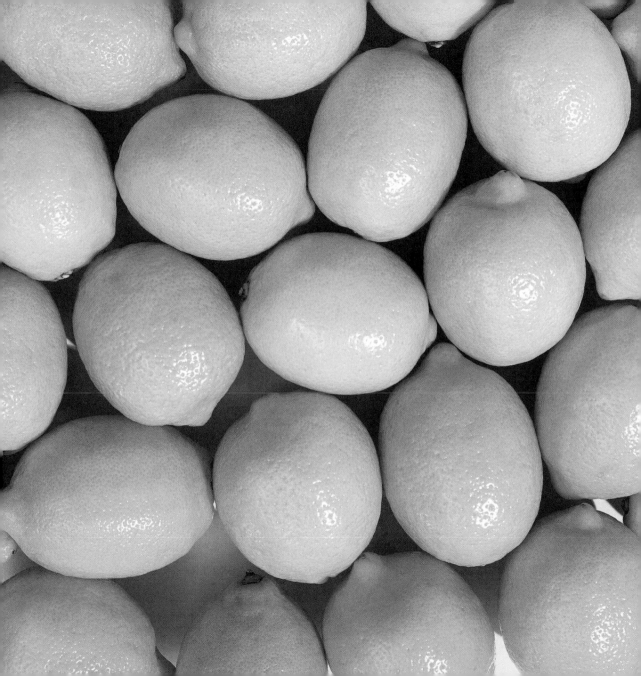

Macrophages are powerful defenders of the body against hostile invaders. They render them ineffective by disintegrating them. Macrophages swallow some parts and attach others to the outside of their cell wall in order to communicate to the secondary defensive cells the appearance of the enemy.

also hidden in our food and swallowed as we eat.

Each part of the body, no matter how tiny, is under constant attack—and in many cases the invaders succeed in leaping past the first barrier, which is the immune system.

The battle against pathogens

Intruders are detected early by a well-functioning immune system and quickly removed. Phagocytes, or macrophages, constantly patrol the body's tissue in search of these uninvited guests, and attack them as soon as they are encountered. The macrophages, our first line of defense, are assisted by the T-lymphocytes. This means that intruders which have managed to penetrate deeper into the organism are also successfully removed. If, during the first line of defense, additional phagocytes attack the intruders, the T-lymphocytes organize what can be described as a targeted defense, in which the entire immune system joins. In this, the T-lymphocytes are assisted by the B-lymphocytes. These form antibodies, which attack their targets in a direct manner, attaching themselves to the intruders and enveloping them. In this manner the intruders are prevented from moving about. Unable to flee from the phagocytes, they are effectively rendered harmless.

T-lymphocytes are also the "archive" of the immune system. They have a memory that stores information about all known attackers for life. When new intruders attempt to penetrate, "files" are created on them, so that they can be immediately recognized and destroyed when next they try to invade.

Danger from within

The line of defense operates in a similar fashion for internal pathogens. This is the case, for example, with cancer cells. These are actually normal body cells that have mutated and are therefore able to multiply indefinitely. Some, however, are not recognized by the body's defense system, because they camouflage themselves and take on the appearance of healthy cells. In such cases a tumor is allowed to grow unchecked. A stable immune system, however, is almost impossible to fool.

Strengthening the Immune System

The yellow fruit contains many substances that promote a healthy immune system.

Vitamin C and bioflavonoids work as a team

Vitamin C counteracts weaknesses in the body's defenses, assisted in this task by bioflavonoids. In addition, the bioflavonoids help to maintain a high vitamin C level in individual body cells. This results in vitamin C deposits throughout the entire body—millions of "gas stations" for the cells of the immune system, which require vitamin C for their work just as much as your car needs gas to drive. Without vitamin C the defense cells would be helpless against intruders and growing cancer cells.

Vitamin C and the fight against free radicals

Macrophages use free radicals in their struggle against pathogens, although the same free radicals are otherwise harmful to the organism. When macrophages, patrolling the body, encounter free radicals, they swallow them and lock them in. There, the free radicals move around like ping-pong balls in a

It is well known that stress and depression weaken the immune system. But it is also true that normally healthy behavior, like physical exercise or sunbathing, can lower the body's resistance if carried to excess.

When you eat lemons or other vitamin C sources, the body's level of this vitamin rises quickly but also declines soon after reaching its peak. To keep the level relatively high and constant, you should take in vitamin C at fairly short and regular intervals.

Most animals have it easier than we do: their bodies actually produce vitamin C. Other than us, only some monkey species, birds, fish and guinea pigs have to supply themselves with the necessary amounts through their diet.

contained space, bouncing from wall to wall. However, when the macrophages encounter a pathogen, they swallow it too and expose it to the ammunition of the free radicals within, which quickly destroy the pathogen by breaking it down into smaller pieces and rendering it harmless.

To protect themselves and their own walls against the free radicals inside, the macrophages need vitamin C. If the vitamin C concentration in the macrophages drops below a certain limit, the defense forces are weakened until they perish. When many macrophages experience this fate, the body's first line of defense is seriously weakened.

Supporting the lymphocytes

The important influence of vitamin C on lymphocytes, the body's second line of defense, has been demonstrated in recent medical studies. Lymphocytes too have high vitamin C levels. When the lymphocytes are challenged and must fight against pathogens, they go into high gear, during which vitamin C is used up more rapidly. If a critical level is not maintained and a vitamin C deficiency occurs, the lymphocytes literally become paralyzed, growing increasingly weaker and ineffective until they perish from the shortage of vitamin C. Should this occur, the second line of defense in the body is weakened to such a degree that the pathogens can do their worst.

Keep Fit with the Lemon Cure

To strengthen your immune system, you should take a six-week lemon cure twice a year. It is recommended that you do so in fall and spring. In fall, this will help prevent susceptibility to colds before the cold and wet season begins. In spring, the cure will bring new energy and prepare pale skin for the strong summer sun. However, you can also use the cure whenever you have the feeling that your immune system could use a boost. For the cure you will require 6 lemons per day and a 3-ounce (100 ml) drop bottle from the pharmacy. The bottle should be made of brown glass to protect the lemon juice from exposure to light.

The immune system knows from birth what pathogens look like. This information is stored in the thymus gland, which is the size of your fist and sits above the heart and behind the sternum.

The lemon cure

Add the juice of 1 lemon, together with 1 tablespoon (15 ml) lemon vinegar (see page 89), to a glass of lukewarm water and sip with breakfast.

1. Cut 1 lemon in half and peel a half so that the white skin remains attached to the flesh of the fruit. Slice and eat with breakfast. Save the second half until evening. To preserve the second half, brush the cut surface with lemon vinegar.

2. Press the juice of 3 more lemons and put into a drop bottle, adding 2 tablespoons (30 ml) lemon vinegar. The lemon vinegar supplies you with important minerals and trace elements and also preserves the vitamin C in the lemon juice. Take 15 to 20 drops every hour throughout the day, until the entire mixture has been consumed by nightfall. Please ensure that you keep to the schedule of hourly drops!

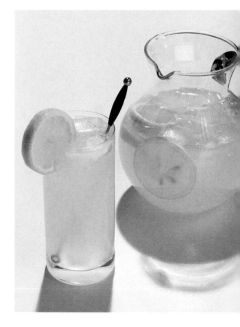

3. Take the sixth lemon and prepare and drink the juice-vinegar-water mixture as in the morning. Eat the second half of the lemon you cut at breakfast (preparation as described for breakfast).

4. Rinse drop bottle with hot water (no detergent) before refilling the next day.

Treating Illnesses from A to Z

Never apply lemon oil before sunbathing on unprotected skin, because all lemon oils photosensitize the skin, which can lead to skin discoloration or eczema.

Lemons deliver many nutrients that protect against or alleviate ailments. Lemons may be used internally as well as externally. Regardless of whether you use lemons in the form of tea or juice, masks or poultices, or in the bath—take advantage of the lemon power pack as a natural healing agent!

Notes on the Use of Lemons

• Rubbing lemon oil or lemon juice preparations into the skin as well as drinking lemon juice and eating the fruit are not appropriate for children under two years of age. Their skin and digestive system are still too delicate to handle it. In older children these applications should be undertaken with care.

• Like all essential oils, lemon oil is a highly concentrated plant extract. Because of its strength it is used sparingly; in most cases a few drops will suffice. It should never be applied to skin or mucous membranes in undiluted form. For full or partial baths, lemon oil is carefully blended with some honey or cream, because this helps to dissolve it better in the bathwater and prevents the droplets from floating to the surface.

- When lemon juice comes into contact with inflamed skin or an open wound, there is often an uncomfortable burning sensation. However, this tends to disappear after a short while.
- For all applications requiring the use of the outer lemon peel, one should use organic lemons purchased in a health food store. This avoids exposure to the harmful chemicals with which commercial lemons are treated. The best choice always is to buy untreated, organic lemons.

Acne

Causes and symptoms

Acne is a chronic skin ailment that predominantly affects adolescents prior to or during puberty—mostly on the face, neck, middle of the chest, shoulders and upper back. Increased production of hormones, in particular testosterone, leads to increased secretions of the sebaceous glands in the skin. At the same time, the gland exit on the skin's surface is blocked, and pockets form beneath the skin. These pockets begin to swell, getting larger and larger and searching for a way through the skin.

At first, all that is visible is a small pimple or tiny black dot. Frequently, these spots become infected within a matter of days, turning red and itchy. If scratched, they burst open and the infectious substances are released onto the surrounding skin. The acne begins to spread, and the characteristic acne pimples develop. Scratching aggravates the infections, which sometimes leave unsightly scars once they are healed.

In the past, people believed that chocolate or spicy foods would aggravate acne. Nowadays, dermatologists believe it is unnecessary to warn against sweets or to advocate special diets.

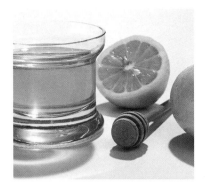

Even skin with acne needs protection against the weather and should not be cleansed too rigorously. You should avoid face lotions with high alcohol content and only treat the infected areas.

Using lemons to treat acne

RINSING WITH LEMON-HONEY WATER

Preparation: Boil 1 quart (1 l) tap water to sterilize it. Let the water cool to 105 degrees Fahrenheit (40ºC). Now dissolve 2 tablespoons (30 ml) of honey in it and add the freshly pressed juice of 1 lemon. *Application:* Wash the areas affected by acne with the lemon-honey water. Be very careful as you do so and make sure that the pimples don't burst in the process. The application should be repeated twice daily, ideally in the morning and the evening.

LEMON/EVENING PRIMROSE OIL FOR SKIN CARE

Preparation: For the oil mixture you will need 1½ ounces (50 ml) jojoba oil, 15 drops pure lemon oil and 15 drops evening primrose oil. Add the other two oils to the jojoba oil and blend well. *Application:* After each treatment with lemon-honey water, massage the lemon/evening primrose oil into the skin in the morning and at night. Use small, gentle circular movements and continue to do so for 5 or 10 minutes. It is important to take this much time (the longer, the better) because the oil should penetrate right into the sebaceous glands. There, it will slow down the activity of the gland and control infection thanks to its disinfecting properties. Let the oil continue to act for some 10 minutes after you finish with the massage and then gently remove any remaining oil on the skin surface with a clean paper towel. To begin with, the excess oil will be quite voluminous, because only a little of it will be able to penetrate into the skin and the glands. However, with each application more of the oil will penetrate. Carry out the massage for a skin cure that should last 3 to 4 weeks.

Bronchitis

Causes and symptoms

There are two types of bronchitis, acute and chronic. The symptoms are the same: a heavy, sometimes painful cough, and white or yellowish sputum as a result of excessive mucus production in the bronchial system. While these symptoms abate after one or two weeks in acute bronchitis, the chronic variety is very hard to get rid of and may flare up again and again over a period of months.

Both types of bronchitis are mainly caused by a virus, such as the rhino virus that causes influenza, and in rarer cases by bacteria. Chronic bronchitis can be aggravated by environmental factors or heavy smoking, which damage the bronchial mucus and make it more susceptible to infections caused by viruses or bacteria.

Dust and dry air aggravate the symptoms of bronchitis. Going for a walk if the air is moist as well as placing bowls of water on the radiators during the colder seasons reduce the stress on the lungs.

Using lemons to treat bronchitis

INHALATION WITH LEMON OIL

Bring 3 cups (750 ml) water to a boil and then let it cool to a temperature where it is still steaming but is comfortable to inhale. (Caution: inhalations with boiling hot water can easily lead to burns in the respiratory tract or on the face.) Before inhaling, add 1 teaspoon (5 ml) salt and 5 drops lemon oil. Inhale 3 times a day until the water has cooled and no more steam rises from it.

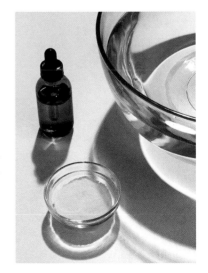

LEMON COUGH SYRUP WITH OLIVE OIL

Blend 3½ oz. (100 ml) freshly squeezed lemon juice and 3½ oz. (100 ml) olive oil. Mix well and take 1 teaspoon (5 ml) every hour. The slight burning sensation in the throat will soon settle.

LEMON SYRUP FOR COUGHING FITS

The antiviral and antibacterial effect of lemons helps to accelerate the healing of bronchitis. In addition, lemon syrup relaxes the bronchial tubes, thereby helping to diminish painful coughing fits, especially during the night.

Place 2 lemons into a pot filled with water, so that they are fully submerged. Place on low heat—approximately 120 degrees Fahrenheit (50°C)—for 10 minutes. The water must not boil, because this would cause the lemons to burst open. Remove the lemons after 10 minutes and squeeze out the juice. Add 3 teaspoons (15 ml) glycerin (obtainable from your pharmacy) to the lemon juice and 9 oz. (250 g) honey, another proven home remedy to soothe coughing. Blend well and your syrup is ready. Take 1 teaspoon (5 ml) before bedtime and another teaspoon should a coughing fit occur in the middle of the night.

CRESS SALAD WITH LEMON

Indian cress or nasturtium is an old healing plant, originating in Peru. It is now available almost year-round. Its leaves contain benzyl-mustard oil, which acts like a mild antibiotic. Salad made with cress and dressed with the juice of a freshly squeezed lemon and some olive oil helps to heal bronchitis when it is caused by bacteria.

LICORICE ROOT/THYME TEA WITH LEMON

The ingredients in licorice root, above all the flavonoids liquiritigenine and liquirititine, ease the cramps in the respiratory system caused by bronchitis, promote expectoration and have a general antibiotic function. The essential oil thymol in thyme also promotes relaxation in the bronchial system and simultaneously kills off any pathogens.

Pour 1 cup (250 ml) boiling water over 1 teaspoon (5 ml) licorice root and 1 teaspoon (5 ml) thyme, let it steep for 5 minutes and pour through a sieve. When the liquid has cooled to body temperature, stir in 1 tablespoon honey and the juice of 2 lemons. Drink 3 cups daily.

Cankers (Mouth Sores)

Causes and symptoms

Cankers are small oval growths on the mucous membrane in the mouth; they can occur throughout the oral cavity and on the tongue. They are usually light to dark gray in the middle, and surrounded by a red ring. Statistics indicate that every fifth person is likely to have cankers at least once in their lifetime, most frequently between the ages of ten and forty. Women are more commonly affected than men. The symptoms of cankers are extremely unpleasant, even painful—especially when they come into contact with something, during eating for example. Cankers are predominantly caused by a virus. They can also result from damage to the mucous membrane in the mouth, caused by brushing one's teeth or biting the delicate membrane inside the mouth, for example. Outbreaks are common when the immune system is weakened for one reason or another, such as when the person affected is already fighting off another illness or when he or she is under a lot of stress. Cankers will generally heal on their own within a week or two.

Medical investigations of cankers (mouth sores) connected with thrush have found bacteria (streptococci), which led to the suspicion that occasionally they might be the source of the infection.

Using lemons to treat cankers

The antibacterial and antiviral properties of lemons have been proven in many different instances. So, they can also help to

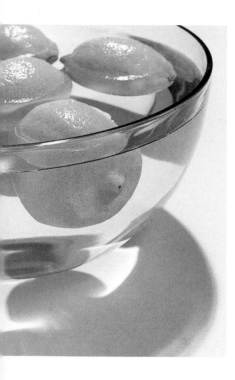

accelerate the healing process in the case of cankers. To achieve this, you should mix the juice of a freshly squeezed lemon into a glass of lukewarm water and rinse the oral cavity with this solution. Do this at least three times a day. You should be aware that when you do this for the first time, there will be a strong burning sensation when the lemon juice mixture comes into contact with the cankers. However, the more frequently you use it, the less burning there will be—and it is also easier to tolerate if you consider that the cankers will heal much more quickly as a result of the rinsing.

Cellulite

Causes and symptoms

A study in Germany revealed that nearly 50 percent of all women in that country suffer from it to some degree: cellulite, the orange-peel skin on the upper thighs and buttocks.

There's no way to predict who will develop cellulite. Young and slim or older and overweight—anyone may be affected. Cellulite is a hereditary change in the connective tissue. Female connective tissue is more elastic than male connective tissue by nature, and therefore better able to stretch. Moreover, a woman's skin is structured so as to store more fat. Both factors play a role in the development of cellulite. However, in addition to fat deposits in the skin, cellulite also occurs in skin with higher levels of water retention and toxins.

THE CELLULITE TEST

It is easy to determine how advanced the cellulite is by applying a pinch test. Pinch the skin on the upper thigh between thumb and index finger, then release.

• If all you see are slight dimples, which disappear on their own after a few seconds, then the changes in the tissue are still in their early stages.

• If the dimples remain visible for a longer period of time and are even visible on an extended leg without pinching, then the cellulite is more advanced.

• If the dimples are also visible while sitting and if the skin hurts when pinched, then there is pronounced cellulite.

Using lemons to treat cellulite

The essential oil of the lemon has tissue-strengthening properties and can therefore contribute to the restoration of weakened connective tissue.

MASSAGE WITH LEMON OIL

Simply mix a few drops of lemon oil with 1 tablespoon (15 ml) jojoba oil and massage into the areas affected by cellulite in the morning and at night.

SKIN-REGENERATING LEMON CELLULITE OIL

Add 15 drops lemon oil to 1½ oz. (50 ml) jojoba oil and 10 drops each of nightshade and cypress oil. You can use the anti-cellulite oil every day—to regenerate the skin, for general skin care and to strengthen the tissue.

Extreme diets tend to aggravate cellulite because the connective tissue, which is already weakened, gets even thinner, whereas the prominent fat cells continue to bulk up anyway.

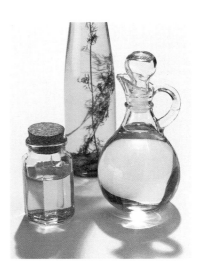

For the long term, in addition to external measures, one should change one's eating habits. The central elements of the diet should be fruit and vegetables high in vitamin C, lean protein from fish, meat, soy products and legumes, and vegetable oils with essential fatty acids.

The rhino virus looks like a porcupine curled into a ball, or a ball with millions of "spikes" sticking out. These viruses are only one ten-thousandth of a millimeter in size. About a thousand billion would fit on the head of a pin.

CELLULITE TEA

Since cellulite is also caused by increased water retention and slack in the tissue, it is important to combine the external treatment with an internal one. You will need 3½ oz. (100 g) stinging nettle leaves, 1¼ oz. (50 g) dandelion root and 1¼ oz. (50 g) spiraea. Take 3 teaspoons (15 ml) of this tea mixture, steep in boiling water for 10 minutes, pour through a sieve and add the juice of 1 lemon for each cup of tea. Drink 2 cups each day for a minimum of 6 weeks.

Colds

Causes and symptoms

Colds are caused by rhino viruses. In contrast to the influenza virus, they are quite harmless, since the cold tends to abate after two weeks by itself. Nevertheless, a cold is still a bothersome and uncomfortable thing. The rhino virus attacks the mucous membranes in the human respiratory system. Once they achieve their goal, these viruses trigger the characteristic cold symptoms: fever, stabbing pain in the head, sore joints, a scratchy throat, cough and runny nose.

Infection by rhino virus

The rhino virus is spread by droplets carried in the air we breathe. In addition, the virus lurks on door handles, phone receivers, pens, etc., and also takes advantage of our friendly custom of shaking hands, during which process it leaps from one person to the other. Once a virus has reached the mucous membrane of the respiratory system, it seeks out one individual cell, whose envelope it pierces with one of its "thorns." On the very first day of infection, the virus penetrates the cell and takes hold there. The virus opens and releases its hereditary information. This forces the mucous membrane cell to continually produce more viruses. On the second day a huge invasion army of rhino viruses is ready to attack the entire respiratory system. The immune system tries immediately to flush out the enemy. The mucous membranes swell and produce more secretions. The patient suffers from a runny nose.

The virus, meanwhile, simply moves on to other mucous cells and forces them to produce more backup. The intruders have the advantage, which the immune system must catch up to. More and more mucous membrane cells die and release thousands of new viruses. The runny nose gets worse, cough and fever may set in—and now the patient is suffering from a full-blown cold.

Using lemons to treat colds

Despite modern pharmaceutical know-how, the medication currently available to fight off the rhino virus is effective only to a limited degree, as various studies have shown. With the power of lemons you will be able to fight off the rhino virus at least as quickly and successfully as with medication. And you will be using a completely natural method, without chemicals that burden the human body. During a cold, the healing power of lemons acts in two ways:

• internally, by supplying urgently required vitamin C to the defense cells, which need the vitamin to perform the tasks we described earlier;

• and externally, through application of its antiviral properties to

If you have a cough, drink plenty of fluids. Most recommended are blackcurrant juice and sea buckthorn juice with lemon.

The home remedy of rinsing your nose dates back to the time when nose drops and nose sprays did not exist. In light of new findings, however, which reveal that the long-term use of some of these medications can damage the mucous membranes of the nose, nose rinses are making a comeback. Even the repeated daily use of nasal rinses over a prolonged period of time does no harm and has no deleterious side effects.

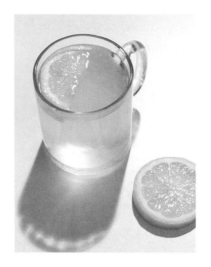

the virus sitting directly on the surface of the mucous membrane in the throat and nose.

A LEMON CURE TO BOOST THE IMMUNE SYSTEM

At the very first sign of a cold, such as a scratchy throat or runny nose, you should immediately supply your body with additional vitamin C by means of a lemon cure in order to boost the immune system, so that the virus doesn't even have a chance to multiply. Drink the freshly squeezed juice of 1 lemon in a glass of lukewarm water every 2 hours. You can further increase the effectiveness by adding 1 tablespoon of lemon vinegar (see page 90) to the beverage twice a day. If the taste is too sour, add honey.

GARGLING WITH LEMON FOR A SORE THROAT

Add the juice of 1 lemon and 1 teaspoon (5 ml) of salt to 1 cup (250 ml) lukewarm water. Gargle 3 times a day for 1 minute. The initial burning sensation will soon diminish.

THROAT DROPS WITH LEMON OIL

Rub 1 sugar cube against the skin of an organic lemon. The essential oil in the peel will be absorbed into the sugar. Suck on several such sugar drops throughout the day.

NOSE RINSE WITH LEMON JUICE

A nose rinse with lemon juice kills off the virus that causes colds and supplies essential minerals to the mucous membrane, keeping it elastic and moist. Your nose will clear up again and you will be able to breathe freely.

Add 1 tablespoon (15 ml) of freshly squeezed lemon juice and

1 pinch of salt to 1 glass of lukewarm water. Hold the glass up to one nostril, close the other nostril with your finger and inhale the liquid through the open nostril. Hold it for a short while, blow it out, then repeat on the other side. Even though this process may be uncomfortable at first due to a tingling sensation in the nose, you will soon become used to it and—most important—will quickly notice a marked improvement in your breathing.

LEMON LEG WRAP TO LOWER FEVER

A leg wrap—wrapping the calves of the legs—is a proven home remedy for lowering fever. The effectiveness is increased even further if lemon oil is used.

Add 8 drops of lemon oil, mixed with 1 tablespoon (15 ml) of cream, to 2 cups (500 ml) cold water. Mix well and soak a linen cloth in the mixture. Squeeze out excess liquid and wrap the cloth around both calves. Now add several layers by means of a large bath towel or two smaller towels. You can remove the wrap after approximately 5 minutes. Always apply to both calves at the same time, at least 3 times a day, until the fever has decreased.

Corns

Causes and symptoms

Over the course of an average lifetime we take more than 300 billion steps; our feet walk a staggering 75,000 miles (120,000 km). Despite this important function, many people select their footwear with little consideration for health. The result: nine out of ten people suffer from one foot ailment or another. Corns are among the most common complaints.

The immune system can produce antibodies only seven days after infection. The antibodies identify the viruses, kill them and encase them in a kind of slime. The yellowish discharge from the nose and the phlegm from coughing expel them from the body.

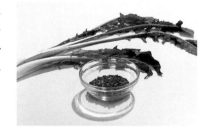

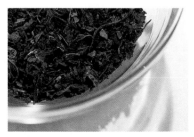

Corns tend to recur at the same spots. After treating a corn, you should protect the affected toe for a while against pressure with a special perforated Band-Aid.

If shoes are too tight, a callus forms at the pressure points, and this callus gradually grows into a corn. A corn "cone" forms at the center of the callus, growing deep into the skin and causing pain.

Using lemons to treat corns

A LEMON POULTICE

Lemon poultices applied overnight are a proven home remedy for corns and their preliminary stage, calluses. Place a slice of lemon approximately $\frac{1}{20}$" to $\frac{1}{5}$" (1–5 mm) thick onto the corn, bandage and fasten. Repeat this application until the corn regresses.

DABBING WITH LEMON OIL

Dabbing the affected area with the essential oil of the lemon accelerates the healing process of corns or callused skin. In addition to the nightly lemon poultice, massage 1 to 2 drops of lemon oil daily into the affected area. Take care to use the undiluted oil only on the callused area and to leave the surrounding skin untouched. Use a cotton ball or a Q-Tip instead of your finger to apply the oil.

Additional measures

• Remember that your shoe size increases as you get older. If you used to wear a size 6, you may need a size 6½ or even size 7 a few years later.

• To prevent pressure on the toes, each shoe should be at least $\frac{3}{5}$" (1½ cm) longer than the foot. The toes should not rub against the uppers and must have enough room to wiggle.

• Pointed shoes crowd the toes and over time will even cause deformations of the foot. A rounded form is much better. Soft leather is preferable to harder materials.

• Purchase a new pair of shoes only after you have tried the fit in the late afternoon or evening and made sure that they are comfortable. Try on the shoes and walk around the store; you won't be able to determine if the shoes pinch while you're sitting down. And always try both shoes.

• Wear flat shoes with flat soles as often as possible. High heels transfer too much of the body weight onto the ball of the foot and the toes, and this area of the foot is much more sensitive than the heel.

If a shoe does not fit properly or chafes somewhere, ask a shoemaker for help. He or she can stretch and soften the shoe, for instance at the heel.

Diarrhea

Causes and symptoms

Diarrhea is the result of an intestinal infection usually caused by bacteria, more rarely by a virus, and occasionally by both at the same time. The body tries to get rid of these pathogens by excreting extremely loose feces, which consists of up to 90 percent water, literally flushing the intruders out.

Lemon juice has proven itself even as a disinfectant against cholera bacteria. It is also an excellent treatment for diarrhea.

Using lemons to treat diarrhea

Lemon juice

When suffering from diarrhea, drink the juice of a freshly squeezed lemon in a large glass of water 3 to 5 times a day. This will kill off the pathogens. In southern countries, germs that cause diarrhea may also be contained in tap water. All water should therefore be brought to a boil first and then cooled. For preven-

Tip: In order to stimulate healing and the regeneration of the skin in cases of eczema, treat the lesions with lemon and afterwards massage some drops of evening primrose oil into the affected area.

tion, 1 to 2 tablespoons (15 to 30 ml) of lemon juice should be taken before every meal.

Eczema

Causes and symptoms

Eczema—a superficial skin infection—may be the result of an allergic reaction, for example to food or medication, or a reaction to external irritants such as chemicals, cleaning agents and similar materials. Doctors at the dermatological clinic in Innsbruck, Austria, have discovered that even dish detergent can cause skin to break out. Studies showed that as little as one teaspoonful (5 ml) of detergent per 2½ gallons (10 l) could severely irritate sensitive skin.

Eczema usually begins with a strong urge to scratch the affected skin area, followed by redness. Later, small blisters will form, which ooze and then crust over.

Using lemons to treat eczema

LEMON WRAP

Add 8 drops lemon oil to 1 cup (250 ml) lukewarm water. To ensure that it blends and is evenly distributed throughout the water, mix the oil thoroughly with 1 tablespoon (15 ml) liquid honey first. Honey too has an anti-inflammatory effect and thus strengthens the healing power of the lemon. Soak a linen cloth in the liquid, squeeze out excess fluid gently and place the cloth on the affected areas for 20 minutes. Repeat this treatment 2 or 3 times per day. The lemon wraps will prevent skin infection on the one hand and also quickly counteract the overwhelming urge to scratch.

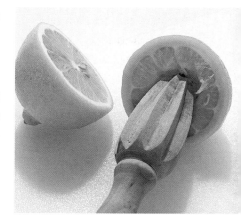

Pure lemon juice can also help to heal minor skin infections quickly. Simply apply a few drops directly onto the affected areas and gently spread it. You may experience a slight burning sensation during the first few minutes.

Gingivitis

Causes and symptoms
If the gums are dark red or if red areas develop where the gum meets the tooth, the first signs of an inflammation of the gums (gingivitis) are present. If this inflammation is well advanced, it will be accompanied by severe pain and bleeding during brushing.

Traces of sugar and carbohydrates that remain attached to the teeth between meals offer an ideal breeding ground for bacteria, which quickly multiply and form plaque. What begins as a soft deposit quickly hardens within a matter of days into a plaque through contact with saliva. The gum begins to swell and separate from the root of the tooth.

Into this pocket bacteria that cause gingivitis can now enter. The inflammation penetrates more deeply and causes the gum to recede even further. In the advanced stages the gum will no longer hold the tooth (a sign of periodontitis). It begins to feel loose and will eventually fall out unless counter-measures are taken.

According to the Canadian Dental Association, 90 percent of Canadians will develop gum disease at some time in their lives. The American Dental Association calls it the U.S.'s number-one oral health issue.

Using lemons to prevent or treat gingivitis

LEMON RINSE

Pour the freshly squeezed juice of 1 lemon into a glass of luke-warm water. Take a mouthful at a time and rinse thoroughly for at least 1 minute.

The lemon juice will kill bacteria, and the acid it contains helps to dissolve the plaque and firm up the gums. Rinse every time you brush your teeth, after the brushing. The tooth enamel will receive a protective coating from the toothpaste, thus protecting it from the lemon acid.

Gout

Causes and symptoms

There are literally millions of people in North America who suffer from gout attacks every now and then: the joints ache and, in the advanced stage, so-called gout knots will form. Gout is a hereditary metabolic disorder. Nevertheless, predisposition alone is not enough to bring on an attack of gout. Only when other conditions combine with the hereditary factor to raise the uric acid levels in the body will gout ensue. When too much of this acid is present in the bloodstream, tiny crystals form, which are deposited in the joints. With each movement their sharp edges rub against the inner skin or cartilage, causing inflammation and pain.

In 60 to 70 percent of all cases the first attack of gout is experienced as sudden, severe pain in the articular bone of the large toe. The skin around the joint is so taut that even the smallest of movements will trigger a sharp pain. Redness and fever often accompany the pain.

What causes increased uric acid levels

High uric acid levels can be caused by:

• *Poor kidney function:* The ability of the kidneys to excrete uric acid from the body has been compromised. This can be the result of any one of a number of kidney ailments or excessive alcohol consumption. When alcohol is metabolized, lactic acid is produced, which hinders uric acid excretion by the kidneys. The same situation can occur due to severe dieting and fasting, which promote excessive production of lactic acid in the intestine.

• *Medication:* Medication to drain water out of the body (prescribed for some people suffering from heart disease), insulin, a number of antibiotics, medication for rheumatism, or an overdose of vitamin B can raise the uric acid level.

• *Poor diet:* Certain foods that contain high levels of purine, for example some fish, legumes and yeasty foods, can also trigger gout. Purine is a protein substance that is transformed into uric acid during digestion. In this manner it can contribute to increased acid concentrations if the kidneys are unable to excrete it quickly enough.

Using lemons to treat gout

The first step is to reduce the body's production of uric acid by means of a diet that contains as little purine as possible. People suffering from gout should avoid the following foods and take meals prepared with lemons as often as possible:

Bad breath, or in severe cases halitosis, is often caused by organic dysfunction: tonsillitis, changes in the mucous membranes of the mouth because of blood disease, slowed saliva flow, bronchitis, inflammation of the stomach lining, and functional disorders of the liver or kidneys.

- meat: offal, meat extracts, veal, bacon
- poultry: turkey, goose
- fish: salmon, mackerel, trout, cod, herring, sardines
- vegetables: peas, beans, lentils, asparagus
- yeast products: baked goods, beer

LEMON JUICE

In addition to a diet low in purine, lemon juice is proven to prevent gout attacks. It stimulates the formation of calcium carbonate in the body. This substance neutralizes acids in the body, including the uric acid that is responsible for gout.

After each meal, drink the freshly squeezed juice of 1 lemon in a glass of lukewarm water.

Halitosis

Causes and symptoms

Some estimates suggust that as many as 60 million people in the United States alone suffer from halitosis. This may be caused by changes in the mouth, throat, nose or stomach region. If the symptoms continue over a long period of time, one should check whether or not an organic cause is the trigger. Often, poor dental health is the problem.

Using lemons to freshen your breath

Lemons help to freshen breath affected by specific spices, alcohol, cigarettes or poor self-cleansing of the throat area as a result of insufficient salivation.

MOUTH RINSE

Thoroughly rinse your mouth several times a day with the freshly squeezed juice of 1 lemon in a glass of water.

LEMON SLICES

Chew on a slice of lemon after every meal.

Hangover

Causes and symptoms

Your head hurts, your throat is dry, everything is painful and slow—the whole world seems to be against you. Nearly everyone has experienced these symptoms after partying all night long. Alcohol, of course, is the cause of a hangover. In the bloodstream the alcohol is transported from the stomach into every single cell in our body. In the brain it quickly develops its intoxicating effect, which camouflages any unpleasantness at first. However, when the metabolism sets in to digest the drug, the brain cells experience an oxygen deficiency, and this is the cause of our sore head the morning after.

In addition, alcohol expands the blood vessels, stimulating the kidneys into overdrive—hence the thirst. With excessive alcohol consumption there may be a magnesium deficiency, whose symptoms are nervousness, trembling hands, muscle cramps and insomnia.

A hangover does more than give you a splitting headache: it also damages your skin. A quick look in the mirror after a night of partying will convince you. Lots of non-alcoholic fluids and energetic exercise in the fresh air, however, will soon bring back a healthy color to your face.

Using lemons to treat a hangover

ANTI-HANGOVER DRINK IN THE MORNING

Add the freshly squeezed juice of 4 lemons, 3 tablespoons (45 ml) of lemon vinegar (see page 89) and 1 pinch of salt to 2 cups (500 ml) lukewarm water. Drink on an empty stomach before breakfast. The acid in the lemon juice helps to support and stimulate your stomach function. Lemon vinegar contains an abundance of minerals, among them magnesium. The salt helps to bind the liquid in the body, preventing it from being immediately excreted by the kidneys.

LEMON COFFEE FOR HEADACHES

Add the juice of 1 lemon to a cup of strong black coffee and drink it unsweetened and without milk. If necessary you can repeat this application as described under the section "Headache" (see page 58).

TO ENHANCE THE EFFECTIVENESS OF LEMONS

• Sometimes a hangover can be averted with an athlete's beverage, which is high in minerals and isotones, taken before bedtime. Chinine-containing bitter drinks, such as ginger ale or Bitter Lemon, have also proven effective. However, you must drink at least 3 cups (750 ml). Two teaspoons of evening primrose oil also prevents the worst symptoms from developing in the first place.
• As first aid in the morning, eating several fresh apples on an empty stomach has been shown to be effective.
• Exercise and fresh air stimulate circulation, which helps to

get rid of the toxins and to balance the oxygen deficiency in the brain.

Tip: While painkillers will alleviate headaches and fatigue, they pose an additional burden for the kidneys. Therefore, you should avoid taking them whenever possible. Try to treat your hangover by natural means—that is, with lemon power.

Hay Fever

Causes and symptoms

Approximately 25 percent of the U.S. population suffer from allergies—and more than 15 percent are affected by hay fever. When trees, bushes and grasses begin to flower in spring and early summer, these individuals suffer from runny nose, itchiness and tearing eyes.

The triggers are the pollen allergens, which are perfectly harmless in principle. However, because of a malfunction in the immune system, the organism unnecessarily combats these allergens, and an increased production of antibodies is the result. During this superfluous defense reaction, there is an excessive production of histamine in the body, which causes the unpleasant hay fever symptoms.

Using lemons to treat hay fever

All parts of the lemon contain quercitrin, but it is especially concentrated in the white subcutaneous layer between the peel and the flesh. The human body produces quercetin from this substance, which functions as a natural antihistamine, suppressing the production of new histamine and the excretion of existing histamine.

During the hay fever season, the skin at the elbows of many allergy sufferers is rough. There's an easy remedy: cut a lemon in half, bend one half slightly at the center and simply place it over the elbow for ten minutes, like a little hat. Repeat frequently and soon the skin will be velvety soft again.

Although quercetin does not completely remedy the symptoms of hay fever, it certainly reduces their severity.

THE PURE LEMON

Carefully peel 1 lemon, leaving as much of the white part of the peel on the lemon as possible. Three weeks prior to your usual hay fever season, begin eating 2 lemons peeled in this manner each day. If you begin to suffer from hay fever, you can increase the amount. The effectiveness is increased if you take 1 to 2 tablespoons (15 to 30 ml) of honey with each lemon. Honey has a powerful anti-allergenic effect, and its high sugar content sweetens the tart lemon diet.

Headache

Causes and symptoms

Headaches are one of the most common ailments. According to the American Council for Headache Education, 90 percent of men and 95 percent of women have at least one headache per year. The International Headache Association distinguishes three main types of headache:

1. Tension headache, caused by muscle spasm and excessive, one-sided strain in the head and neck area. This headache is concentrated in the forehead and temples. It is usually caused by stress, emotional conflict or poor posture.

2. Cluster headaches predominantly afflict men, in sudden attacks that can last for days or months. These extreme aches are concentrated on one side of the head and, in contrast to migraines, are accompanied by a stabbing or pulling type of pain.

3. The pounding, pulsating migraine pain resides in one side of the head and can last anywhere from several minutes to several days. During a migraine attack there is a dysfunction of the

neuron pathway. This can cause an inflammatory reaction in the brain vessels accompanied by pain, nausea, and neurological dysfunction such as zigzag lines or blurred vision.

Using lemons to treat headaches

LEMON COFFEE

Mix the freshly squeezed juice of 1 lemon into a cup of strong black coffee. Drink it unsweetened and without milk. If the pain does not subside, take up to 3 cups of lemon coffee daily.

Lemon coffee is a great antidote if you are sensitive to changes in the weather.

LEMON PEEL

Peel 1 large organic lemon. There are two ways in which lemon peel can be used for headaches:
• Bend the lemon peel slightly between your fingers, stretching the outer side of the peel. Then rub it against your temples to massage the essential oil into your skin.
• Remove the layer of white skin underneath the peel. Press the inside of the lemon peel against your temples. You will feel a slight burning sensation, but the headache should disappear quickly.

LEMON OIL MIXTURE FOR MIGRAINE

Mix 3½ oz. (100 ml) jojoba oil with 20 drops lemon oil as well as 10 drops each of camomile oil, lavender oil and peppermint oil, and 6 drops rosemary oil. Massage several drops of this mixture into your temples and onto the nape.

It is not advisable to take over-the-counter combination drugs when you have a headache. The interaction of the various substances contained in them can, over time, lead to very severe kidney damage, as Marc de Broe, a nephrologist in Belgium, has found out.

The herpes virus is ten to a hundred times smaller than a bacterium and invades the cells of the body unnoticed. There, it changes the cell metabolism and multiplies. Eventually the host cell is destroyed, breaks open and releases many more viruses, which in turn attack other cells.

Appoximately 90 percent of the population of North America is said to be infected with the herpes virus. That does not mean, however, that all of those infected will show the symptoms.

Herpes

Causes and symptoms

Lip blisters are caused by the herpes virus. Initial contact with the virus generally occurs within the first five years of a person's life. The herpes virus will remain in the body throughout the person's life, but it lies dormant for most of the time. No effective means have been discovered to kill it.

Several factors combine to wake the herpes virus from its slumber and activate it. These may be physical and emotional situations, such as fever, menstruation, injury, infection or strong UV exposure. The symptoms are always the same: at first the patient feels a sensation of tightness in the lip, combined with itchiness and burning. Gradually the infection spreads and blisters form. The blisters will crust over and heal within 6 to 14 days.

Using lemons to treat herpes

DABBING WITH LEMON OIL

Once again the antiviral properties of lemon oil come into play. Place 1 drop of the oil, this time undiluted, on the end of a Q-Tip and dab the blister. Take care not to make any brushing or stroking movements: should the blister break open, you would be spreading the infection.

THE BIG LEMON CURE

At the same time, you should take measures to boost your immune system. The herpes virus doesn't stand a chance if your immune system is strong and healthy. The best approach is to take the big lemon cure described in the chapter "Prevention with the Power of Lemons" (see page 35).

High Blood Pressure (Hypertension)

Causes and symptoms

More than one in three women and nearly every second man over the age of forty suffers from high blood pressure, a dangerous time bomb that can lead to heart attack or stroke in the long term. The most common cause is arteriosclerosis, a narrowing of the arteries due to deposits in the walls of the vessels. Other possible causes of high blood pressure include kidney, gland and heart disease as well as the side effects of medication. However, all these causes combined account for only 5 percent of all high blood pressure patients. In roughly 95 percent of cases it is impossible to determine a cause, despite detailed research. In these situations doctors speak of essential high blood pressure, where the precise cause or causes remain hidden.

Using lemons to treat high blood pressure

LEMON MILK
Add 3 crushed garlic cloves and 1 chopped onion to 1 quart (1 l) cold milk. Slowly bring the milk to a boil and let it stand for 5 minutes. Pour it through a sieve and chill. Add the freshly squeezed juice of 3 lemons and sip throughout the day.

LEMON VINEGAR AND HONEY WATER
Add 2 tablespoons (30 ml) lemon vinegar (see page 89) to 1 glass

A good home remedy for high blood pressure is a "rice day" once a week. On that day eat nothing but rice boiled in water. You can enhance the taste by adding grated apples and lemon juice, but under no circumstances add salt, because that would negate the beneficial diuretic effect.

lukewarm water, then add the freshly squeezed juice of 2 lemons and dissolve 1 tablespoon (15 ml) of honey in the mixture. Honey is rich in magnesium, a vasodilator, thus helping to lower blood pressure. Throughout a long treatment period, drink a glass of this mixture in the morning for breakfast and another at night before bed.

OLIVE LEAF AND HAWTHORN TEA WITH LEMON JUICE

Olive leaves (available at the pharmacy) and hawthorn contain flavonoids, which are effective in the fight against high blood pressure and combine well with the power of the lemon into a tea blend.

Application: The basis for the tea consists of 2 parts olive leaves and 1 part hawthorn leaves. Pour boiling water over 1 heaped tablespoon (15 ml) of this plant mixture. Let the tea steep for 10 minutes and then cool to a lukewarm temperature. Add the freshly squeezed juice of 2 lemons. Drink a cup of this tea–juice blend every day, preferably in the evening before bedtime. Within 3 weeks of starting this treatment you will notice a marked improvement in your blood pressure.

BUCKWHEAT MUESLI WITH LEMON JUICE

Ingredients: 1 dash salt, 1 cup (250 ml) water, 9 oz. (250 g) buckwheat, 2 tbsp. (30 ml) raisins, 2 tbsp. (30 ml) honey, 4 tbsp. (60 ml) cream, 1 lemon

Preparation: Add the salt to the water and bring to a boil. Stir in the buckwheat and simmer on low heat until it forms into a porridge. Cool and mix in the raisins, honey and cream. Press the juice out of one whole lemon and pour over the muesli. Use this

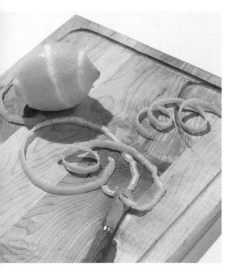

muesli instead of your breakfast toast or afternoon snack as often as possible for improved blood pressure.

Influenza

Causes and symptoms
The influenza virus causes a severe infection of the respiratory tract. For people whose immune system is already weakened, an influenza infection can be fatal. Influenza can also lead to pneumonia and bronchitis, middle ear infections or arrhythmia. These so-called secondary illnesses are caused by other disease germs that attack when the body is weakened by influenza. The secondary infections too can be life-threatening, especially for the elderly and the very young.

Using lemons to treat influenza
Medication can do little in the fight against the flu. The only effective prevention is a vaccination in the fall of each year. Since the virus mutates frequently, the immunity gained from earlier vaccinations no longer offers adequate protection. Therefore, the composition of the vaccine is modified every year.

If a patient has not been vaccinated and is infected by influenza, treatment by a doctor is essential. At this stage, home remedies will not suffice, and the longer a doctor's treatment is postponed, the more dangerous the course of the illness might be.

LEMON CURE
Lemons can prove very effective supplements to and supports for medical treatment, by strengthening the immune system with the

The new flu viruses that appear each year originate in the remote regions of Asia, Siberia and western China. That is where they continually change their appearance, as "old" human viruses get crossed with those of animals. Birds carry them on their long migrations to Europe, whence they quickly spread to North America. When people get infected with these new viruses, the immune system is unable to recognize them as disease carriers because of their altered appearance. That is how the great epidemics start.

Candles scented with lemon oil can help against pesky mosquitoes whether you burn the candles inside the house or on the porch. It is easy to make scented candles yourself. Melt down any leftover candle bits and add a few drops of lemon oil. Take a small flowerpot, plug the hole at the bottom, add a wick and pour in the liquid wax.

natural vitamin C they contain. Apply the lemon cure described for colds (see page 46).

Insect Bites

Causes and symptoms

The arrival of warm weather brings unwelcome guests: mosquitoes and blackflies, hungry for human blood. Their bite is often unpleasant, and sometimes it continues to be bothersome for days. It is red and itchy. The reason for this discomfort is in fact a small infection caused by foreign bodies or chemical substances transferred during the insect bite. The bites of bees, wasps and similar insects are even more painful, because they inject their poison directly into the skin.

Using lemons to treat insect bites

FIRST AID WITH LEMON OIL AND LEMON VINEGAR

If the sting is still in the skin, remove it with tweezers. Massage 1 to 2 drops of lemon oil, mixed with 1 teaspoon (5 ml) of honey, into the skin around the bite. This will prevent infection. Next, add a dash of lemon vinegar to a glass of water (see page 89), soak a handkerchief with the mixture and apply.

THE LEMON AS INSECT REPELLENT

Add 20 drops lemon oil to 1 cup (250 ml) water and spray into the air. Not only does it smell wonderful and fresh, but it will also repel insects. Another proven home remedy is to place a cotton wad soaked in lemon oil next to the bed overnight.

Or run a fresh lemon peel over your skin to disperse the essential oil.

If you're sitting outside in the evening, you can repel insects by applying lemon scent to the skin areas not covered by clothing. Add 10 drops lemon oil to 1½ oz. (50 ml) wheat germ or sunflower oil and rub into skin.

Lack of Concentration

Causes and symptoms
Lack of concentration is a typical symptom of our hectic age. It is often accompanied by nervousness, insomnia, forgetfulness, or learning difficulties in children. Stress, worries in one's professional or personal life, or emotional conflict are the usual triggers for concentration problems.

Using lemons to treat lack of concentration
The psycho-emotional properties of lemon oil can help alleviate lack of concentration or a general sense of low performance; they are also helpful in case of fatigue and even mild depression. At the same time, the oil stimulates brain activity.

Aromatherapy with lemon oil
Add 4 drops lemon oil to a water-filled aromatherapy lamp. In this manner you will breathe away your malaise without even noticing it.

HUMIDIFICATION WITH LEMON OIL
Add 15 drops lemon oil to 2 cups (500 ml) water and spray into

Insects are attracted by scents, whether it is perspiration, perfume, sunscreen, hairspray or even kitchen smells. Allergy sufferers should avoid wearing brightly colored or loose-fitting, flapping clothing. They should also avoid walking barefoot on grass.

Your ability to concentrate suffers if the healthy rhythm between stress and relaxation is broken. More and more people are losing the ability to relax. You can counteract that problem with meditation or techniques such as autogenic training or Jacobson's progressive muscle relaxation.

Most nosebleeds can be stopped by squeezing the nostrils between thumb and index finger and breathing through your mouth.

the air with an atomizer. *Caution:* Avoid letting droplets land on sensitive surfaces, where they could stain!

Nosebleeds

Causes and symptoms
Nosebleeds are generally harmless, caused by some minor injury to the small veins in the septum (the partition between the nostrils), just inside the opening of the nose. The trigger may be a direct impact on the nose or heavy sneezing.

Caution: frequent nosebleeds
If nosebleeds are regular or frequent, a doctor should be consulted to determine if a more severe ailment may be the cause. Different types of blood diseases, high blood pressure, liver damage, tumors and vascular disease may cause nosebleeds.

Using lemons to treat nosebleeds

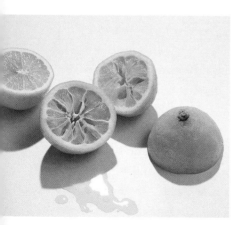

DABBING
Squeeze some juice from a fresh lemon, soak a Q-Tip in it, and dab the inside of your nose gently. The head should be tilted slightly forward, to prevent the blood from flowing into the throat. You can also place a cold compress on the forehead and nape. Lemons have astringent properties. As soon as injured blood vessels come into contact with lemon juice, they contract. The open wound closes and the bleeding stops.

Osteoporosis

Causes and symptoms

Osteoporosis is the most common bone disease in adults. The onset commonly occurs near the sixtieth year and affects mostly women—in fact, nearly one in three women. The tricky aspect is that this is a silent disease, nearly imperceptible at the beginning. There are hardly any symptoms, then suddenly there are painful vertebrae dysfunctions, visible on the outside in the so-called dowager's hump. The cause of the increased brittleness in the bone is a diminution of bone tissue in old age. From the fortieth year onward, our bones lose approximately 1.5 percent of their mass each year. When you multiply this loss by thirty, then at least one-third of the total bone mass is lost by the age of seventy. Women are particularly affected because in menopause their bodies are deprived of the hormone estrogen, which is essential for bone regeneration. When the situation is exacerbated by a calcium deficiency, the bone loss can be severe. The body urgently requires calcium to build up bone mass and to maintain it. Approximately 2.2 pounds (1 kg) of calcium is stored in the human skeleton.

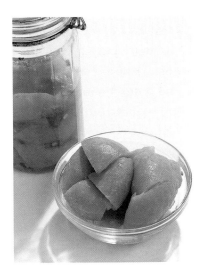

Early prevention of osteoporosis

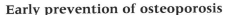

• Because calcium is essential for the body to build bone mass, you should begin by including more calcium-rich foods in your diet, such as milk products, fish, fresh vegetables and herbs, and sea salt. Foods rich in phosphates and oxalic acid, such as meat, cola drinks, spinach, rhubarb and tomato, on the other hand, inhibit calcium absorption in the intestine, and their intake should therefore be reduced.

Osteoporosis sufferers should do special exercises for the spine. It is also important that they do not carry heavy loads, that they keep their back and neck straight while working, and that they acquire an elastic but firm mattress for their bed.

In the case of calcium deficiency, not only does the production of new bone tissue stop, but calcium is taken out of existing bone material in order to continue with all the other metabolic functions that require calcium.

• Lower your alcohol and nicotine consumption, because excessive amounts of these substances can damage the skeleton.

• Ensure that you get sufficient exercise. Regular exercise or calisthenics promotes the regeneration of bone tissue.

Using lemons to prevent osteoporosis

COOKING WITH LEMONS

You can support calcium absorption by using lemons as often as possible in your meal preparation. For example, use lemon vinegar (see page 89) for salad dressing.

LEMON VINEGAR AND LEMON JUICE

Lemon acid plays an important role in helping the body to absorb and use calcium, and thus helps to prevent osteoporosis. Lemon vinegar contains calcium and lemon acid—in other words, both the substance necessary for bone regeneration and the substance that improves its absorption.

Drink 1 glass of warm water with the freshly squeezed juice of 1 lemon and 1 tablespoon (15 ml) of lemon vinegar twice each day, once before breakfast and again before dinner. If you sweeten the drink with 1 tablespoon (15 ml) of honey, you will increase the natural calcium content. People who have an intolerance to lactic acid or another allergy should take the juice of 1 lemon with every meal to compensate for their limited intake of calcium.

Rheumatism

Causes and symptoms

Some 37 million people in the United States are affected by rheumatism to some degree (that's one in seven), and it is estimated that 85 percent of Canadians will be affected by rheumatism by age seventy. "Rheuma" itself isn't really a disease, but a superannuated term for nearly four hundred different diagnoses that can all be collected under the wider term "rheumatism." What they have in common is that they affect our mobility, are linked with pain and can severely restrict our ability to move.

The most common forms of rheumatism

- *Degenerative rheumatism:* One-sided stress on individual joints, for example at the workplace, can lead to severe wear and tear. Nearly 80 percent of all people over the age of sixty suffer from this type, which includes arthritis as well as damage to the discs and vertebrae.
- *Inflammatory rheumatism:* A malfunction of the immune system can cause the defense cells to attack the body's own organism. They attack the inner skin on the joints and cause an inflammation of the joint. In the long term, the delicate tissue is destroyed. Different types of arthritis, Morbus Bechterew (Ankylosing Spondylitis) and chronic polyarthritis fall into this category of diseases that affect several joints simultaneously. Over 2 million patients suffer from this ailment in North America
- *Extra-articular rheumatism:* Here it is the soft tissues and not the joints that are affected: muscles, tendons, bursa, ligaments, nerves or the connective tissue of the subcutis. Constant excessive

Arthritis by itself is painful enough, but it is often accompanied by other afflictions, such as diabetes mellitus, high blood pressure, kidney damage or bladder stones. That is why countermeasures should be taken from the first symptoms and applied consistently.

One of the many theories about the cause of rheumatoid diseases is based on the assumption that excessive acidity in the body is a major catalyst, and that high levels of acidity in the joints and soft tissue crucially influence the progression of the disease and aggravate the pain associated with it.

A balanced diet for arthritis sufferers should include low-fat milk products, lean meat in small portions, lots of fresh fruit and vegetables, pasta, potatoes and, above all, much liquid in the form of fruit juices, coffee and tea.

Warm baths of any kind, including full baths, are counter-indicated for those suffering from inflammatory rheumatoid diseases unless prescribed by a physician, because warmth generally increases acute inflammation.

strain on these soft tissues over extended periods of time can cause cramps and strains that may become chronic. A typical example: tennis elbow.

Using lemons to treat rheumatism

MASSAGE WITH LEMON OIL
Massage the affected area on a daily basis with several drops of lemon oil mixed with 1 tablespoon (15 ml) jojoba oil. This will inhibit inflammation, relax cramps and ease the pain.

HEALING LEMON TEA
Spiraea is rich in salicylic acid compounds such as salicylaldehyde and methyl salicylate, but also in tannic agents and the flavonoid spriaeoside, which together have excellent effects on rheumatic ailments.

Pour 1 cup (250 ml) boiling water over 2 teaspoons (10 ml) spiraea, let steep for 10 minutes and pour through a sieve. Once it is cool enough to drink, add the juice of 1 freshly squeezed lemon to each cup of the tea. Drink 2 cups daily; in case of acute pain, 3 cups daily.

DE-ACIDIFICATION WITH LEMON JUICE
Even though it tastes sour, lemon juice has a powerful alkaline effect in the body and is therefore a natural agent against excess acid, which is in part responsible for rheumatism. Drink the freshly squeezed juice of 1 lemon in a glass of lukewarm water 3 times a day. Double the dosage—that is, the juice of 2 lemons 3 times a day—whenever you are experiencing acute pain.

Spider Veins

Spider veins are common in every second woman over twenty. Men too can be affected, although this is less common. In principle, spider veins are more of a cosmetic than a health issue, because they are harmless. These are expanded, small veins in the upper layer of the skin that become visible as fine blue lines. They most often occur in the cheeks, nose, and upper and lower thighs.

It is still largely unclear how spider veins initially develop. Some evidence suggests that hereditary factors, excessive alcohol consumption, frequent and long sunbathing, as well as the contraceptive pill may play a role.

Using lemons to treat spider veins

LEMON OIL MASSAGE

Lemon oil has vessel-strengthening properties, which also help to strengthen the walls of the expanded veins. Take 2 or 3 drops of lemon oil every day and mix it in a small bowl with jojoba, avocado or almond oil, and massage the affected areas.

REGENERATING LEMON OIL BATH FOR VEINS AND VESSELS

Add 8 drops lemon oil to a bathtub filled with water between 85 and 95 degrees Fahrenheit (30–34°C). Also add 4 drops cypress oil that you have previously blended with 1 tablespoon (15 ml) liquid honey or cream. Soak in the bath for 15 to 20 minutes. When you step out, do not rub your skin vigorously with a towel

Lemon and cypress oil can be added to footbaths too, if only the lower legs have spider veins. Just make sure you adjust the dose accordingly.

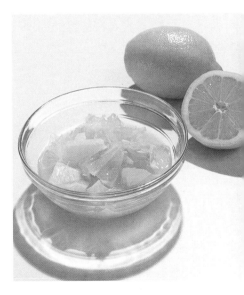

About one person in ten thousand infected with *helicobacter pylori* bacteria will develop stomach cancer. If the infection is diagnosed early enough, there are drugs available that provide very effective treatment, delivering a long-term cure to 90 percent of patients.

but pat it dry instead. Make sure that the temperature does not exceed 95 degrees, otherwise the veins might expand even further.

Stomach Ailments

Causes and symptoms

Food travels through the esophagus to the stomach. There, it is digested with stomach acid, and the stomach muscles contract until the food fragments are split into tiny pieces. Then it travels onward to the small intestine. This process usually occurs without us even noticing it. Sometimes, however, we may have an uncomfortable feeling of being overly full. We say that the meal lies heavy in our stomach. What is really happening is that the stomach muscles aren't working properly, or insufficient amounts of stomach acid are being produced. Consequently, we experience pressure in the stomach or feel the food rising, because it has remained in the stomach for too long without being digested or transported forward.

Long-lasting pain

If you experience discomfort or pain in the stomach region for an entire week without interruption, you must consult a doctor. The cause may be that the bacterium *Helicobacter pylori* has taken hold in the mucous membrane of the stomach. In addition to causing severe lymph ailments, this bacterium may also be responsible for stomach cancer.

Statistically, 50 percent of the world's population is infected with *Helicobacter pylori*. Approximately 30 percent of North

Americans have the bacterium. And in every seventh or eighth person this infection develops into a benign growth in the stomach or duodenum.

Using lemons to treat stomach aches

LEMON JUICE

Drink the freshly squeezed juice of 1 lemon in a glass of lukewarm water with each meal. The lemon acid stimulates the production of stomach acid and the activity of the stomach muscles. A pleasant side effect: lemon juice can also help you lose weight if you take 2 tablespoons (30 ml) with each meal.

Sunburn

Causes and symptoms

Exposure to strong sun, and especially to UV rays, can cause burns in the upper layers of the skin. Individual cells are destroyed, the skin turns red and it burns. Depending upon the severity of the sunburn, the top layer of skin may peel. The actual damage to the skin is often much more severe than is visible to the naked eye. Repeated sunburns increase the risk of skin cancer.

Using lemons to soothe sunburn

SPONGE BATH

Take sponge baths with cold lemon water. To do so, add the freshly squeezed juice of 3 lemons to 2 cups (500 ml) cold water

According to new findings, larger doses of vitamins C and E strengthen the skin's protection against the sun. Results from experiments with volunteers showed that after only one week their skin could take a longer exposure to the sun without reddening. Nevertheless, an effective sunscreen is a definite must.

Especially in early childhood, our tonsils play an important role in the development of the immune system. Tonsillectomy as a treatment for chronic tonsillitis should therefore be considered only when a child has reached school age.

and carefully wash the areas affected by sunburn. The lemon water cools, acts as a disinfectant and helps the skin to heal.

LEMON–HONEY POULTICE

After taking the lemon sponge bath, you should follow with a mild healing poultice. To prepare it you will need 9 oz. (250 g) low-fat cheese curd, 2 tablespoons (30 ml) clear honey and 1 tablespoon (15 ml) lemon juice. Mix all the ingredients and spread the poultice on the affected areas. Rinse with clear water after 15 minutes.

SKIN OIL FOR BURN BLISTERS

First-degree burns can be alleviated with this mixture, which will also help the healing process. Mix 40 drops nightshade oil with 30 drops lemon oil. Massage a few drops several times a day onto the affected area.

Tonsillitis

Causes and symptoms

Most cases of tonsillitis are caused by bacteria (streptococcus); more rarely it is the result of a virus. The tonsils in the back of the throat become red, swollen and covered in small yellow pustules. Symptoms include difficulty swallowing, sore throat and, in advanced cases, fever.

Careful: long-term damage after tonsillitis!

Should the fever rise above 102 degrees Fahrenheit (39°C) during a bout of tonsillitis, or if the illness continues for more than

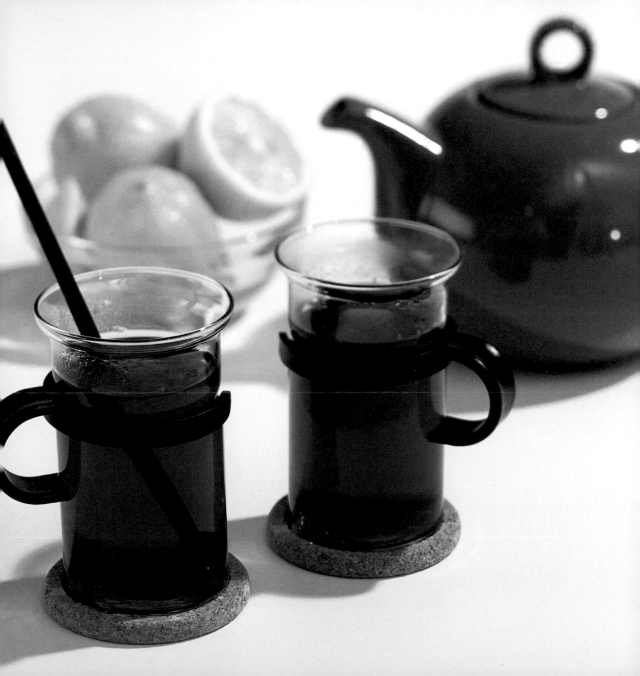

It has been said that spider veins are an early indicator of future varicose veins, but so far we have no evidence of that. Common to both may be a general disposition to weak connective tissue.

a week, it is extremely important to consult a doctor. When tonsillitis doesn't heal fully, there is a danger that the streptococcus can spread throughout the body via the bloodstream. The consequences may be severe kidney damage or a dangerous paralysis of the heart muscle, which could even lead to heart failure in an advanced stage.

Using lemons to treat tonsillitis

GARGLING WITH LEMON JUICE

Gargle every 2 hours for at least 30 seconds with the freshly squeezed juice of 1 lemon. Tilt your head far back to allow the juice to flow into the back of the throat. The antibacterial and antiviral properties of lemon juice will work directly on the pathogens.

You can swallow the juice when you are finished gargling, thereby benefitting from a vitamin C boost and also from the bioflavonoids, both of which help to strengthen the immune system from within.

Varicose Veins

Causes and symptoms

Every fourth man and every second woman suffers from varicose veins. Nearly one in nine adults will experience more or less severe symptoms caused by varicose veins: tension, heavy or swollen legs, a tingling sensation when lying down or sitting, nocturnal cramps in the calves, a pulling sensation and pain. This vein ailment is caused by a dysfunction in the flow of blood as it returns to the heart. Varicose veins occur when this mechanism no longer functions properly because the venous valves are defective at one or more points or no longer close at all. The blood accumulates in the legs and the veins become swollen—a condition that is visible on the outside as thick blue strands. In addition to being unsightly, varicose veins can pose considerable problems and lead to water accumulation in the legs (edema), leg sores that won't heal or even vein inflammations.

Since the walls of veins are for the most part made up of connective tissue, one out of three women will experience problems during the first three months of pregnancy.

The three types of varicose veins

Vein specialists (phlebologists) differentiate between three types of varicose veins that may occur on the legs:

• The thick stem vein that is formed when the defect occurs in the groin. The entire blood from the leg region gathers into a pool in this area and flows back to the heart via the large pelvic vein. In the case of a disorder in the veins and the resulting changes, it can happen that the blood flows back into the legs and gathers there.

• Branched varicose veins can occur on the upper and lower leg if the blood from the stem vein is pushed into the secondary veins located there.

• The smallest type of perforating varicose veins are tiny lateral links between the superficial and lower veins in the legs, and these pose few problems.

Risk factors

• *Genetic predisposition:* In approximately 80 percent of people with varicose veins there is a strong predisposition. However, this alone need not lead to varicose veins. The number of other risk

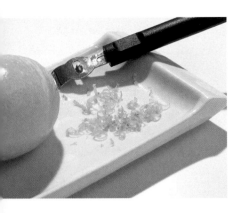

factors that are added to the predisposition will determine whether or not varicose veins will form.

• *Pregnancy:* Hormonal changes in the body of a pregnant woman cause a general weakening in the connective tissue. This is exacerbated as the pregnancy progresses by an increased pressure on the downward veins as a result of the enlarged uterus. However, most varicose veins resulting from pregnancy tend to heal on their own after the baby is born.

• *Contraceptive pill:* Because the pill tricks the body into a state of constant "pregnancy," the female body reacts with the same hormonal changes present during a real pregnancy, thereby potentially weakening the connective tissue.

• *Lack of exercise:* People whose work requires standing for long periods will often develop varicose veins. The pressure of the entire column of blood in the body is brought to bear on the veins in the legs. If this pressure isn't alleviated by the "pumping action" that muscles perform during exercise, the vessels will expand over time. As a result, the venous valves no longer close tight, and widening and varicose veins are the consequence. Too much leg exercise isn't good either, however: soccer players and dancers often suffer from varicose veins.

Using lemons to treat varicose veins

In principle the same applications described under "Spider Veins" (page 71) can be used for varicose veins. When using the lemon oil massage, make sure that you gently massage from bottom to top, that is from the feet upwards, in the direction of the heart.

In addition, there are some other lemon therapies whose vessel-strengthening effects have proven to be useful in preventing or treating varicose veins.

MASSAGE WITH LEMON OIL MIXTURE

Add 6 drops lemon oil to 1½ oz. (50 ml) wheat germ oil and 2 drops each of cypress and juniper oil. Use this mixture daily for a gentle massage of the legs from bottom to top, always in the direction of the heart.

LEMON OIL WRAP

Add 5 drops lemon oil mixed with 1 tablespoon (15 ml) cream to 1 cup (250 ml) warm water. Soak cloths and wrap the affected areas. Leave the wrap on for a minimum of 15 minutes and elevate your legs during this time. The treatment should be repeated on a daily basis.

LEMON OIL FOOTBATH

Mix 6 drops lemon oil, 2 drops cypress oil, 2 drops juniper oil and 2 drops rosemary oil with 1 tablespoon (15 ml) honey. Fill a small tub with warm water (85–93°F / 30–34°C) and add the mixture. Stir well and bathe for 20 minutes. Take daily footbaths.

A lemon oil bath can help reinvigorate the blood vessels and fight varicose veins when the legs feel tired and heavy. For dosage and application, consult the entry under "Spider Veins" (page 71).

CHAPTER 5

Beauty Care with Lemons

The many nutrients and anabolic agents in lemons make them not only a popular choice for home remedies but also a very effective ingredient in natural beauty products. We have collected a few simple recipes for daily skin and hair care, and for the treatment of some minor cosmetic problems. So go ahead and try some, and find out which of the body oils, hair treatments and bath mixtures described here suit you best.

Skin Care

Lemons are a truly magical ingredient for skin care. Lemon creams and oils slow down the aging process; they firm, cleanse and regenerate skin—all in the most natural manner imaginable and with their inimitable fresh scent. This is why the yellow fruit is a popular ingredient in the cosmetics industry, where it is used in many preparations. You can give your skin the same benefit with very little effort and at a fraction of the cost by using homemade preparations.

Oils for face and body

PREPARATION FOR OILY SKIN

Ingredients: 1 ½ oz. (50 ml) cold-pressed jojoba oil, 6 drops lemon oil, 4 drops cypress oil
Application: Blend the jojoba oil with the lemon and cypress oil. Gently massage your face with this mixture every morning and night.

LEMON GRASS–LEMON OIL

Ingredients: 1 cup (250 ml) jojoba oil, 1 cup (250 ml) avocado oil, 2 lemons, 4 stems of fresh lemon grass (available at most greengrocers), 2 tbsp. (30 ml) dried lemon grass (from your herbalist or health food store), 1 bottle made of brown glass with a tightly closing top, 30 drops evening primrose oil
Application: Mix the jojoba oil with the avocado oil and add the fresh peel of the lemons and the squeezed juice. Cut the lemon grass stems into pieces about 1 inch (2–3 cm) in length and place on a chopping board. Crush to release the juice from inside the stems; this alone releases the essential oil of the lemon grass. Add the crushed pieces and the dried lemon grass to the oil mixture.

Place the bottle containing the oil into a water bath for 30 minutes. Leave the bottle open. The water temperature should be between 105 and 120 degrees Fahrenheit (40–50°C). Remove and close tight. Store at room temperature. The bottle should be stored for approximately 1 month to allow the valuable substances in the lemon grass and the lemon to be absorbed into the

Jojoba oil and avocado oil are especially easy on the skin and are therefore most suitable as vehicles in skin care products with essential oils. They rarely turn rancid when stored in dark bottles at room temperature.

Rubbing the affected areas with lemon grass–lemon oil is an excellent treatment for muscle spasms of the lower back, rheumatic inflammations, sprains and bruises. You may use the pure oil, that is, without adding evening primrose oil.

oil. During this time you should shake it slightly every second day.

After 1 month, pour the oil through a linen cloth to strain out the pieces of lemon grass and lemon peel. Now add the evening primrose oil and shake vigorously. The oil can be used for general skin care and to revitalize your skin.

Masks and packs

LEMON MASK FOR WRINKLES

Ingredients: 1 egg yolk, 1 tbsp. (15 ml) jojoba oil, 1 lemon
Application: Blend the egg yolk and jojoba oil. Squeeze the juice out of the lemon and add to the blend. Massage mixture into wrinkles. Leave on for 20 minutes and remove with very cold water.

MASK FOR OILY SKIN

Ingredients: 2 cups (500 ml) water, 5 drops lemon oil, 1 tbsp. (15 ml) cream
Application: Heat the water and add the lemon oil previously mixed with the cream. Soak a linen cloth in the mixture and apply to the skin for 15 minutes.

LEMON AND CHEESE CURD PACK FOR TIRED SKIN

Ingredients: 1¾ oz. (50 g) low-fat cheese curd, 5 drops lemon oil, 2 tbsp. (30 ml) lukewarm water, 1 tbsp. (15 ml) honey
Application: Add the lemon oil to the low-fat cheese curd, then add water and finally the honey. Stir well and apply to skin. Rinse with warm water after 15 to 20 minutes. Gently pat skin dry.

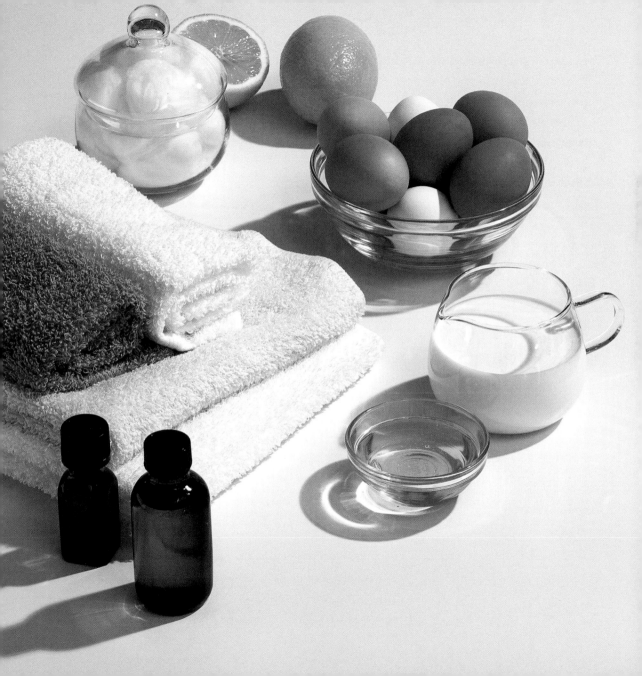

All skin care preparations should always be freshly produced. Please do not save the leftovers! The ingredients spoil easily, and the vitamin C of the lemon loses its potency rapidly when exposed to light and air.

LEMON–BANANA MASK FOR DRY SKIN

Ingredients: 1 ripe banana, 3 drops lemon oil, 1 shot glass each of avocado and jojoba oil, 2 egg yolks, 2 lemons

Application: Squash the banana and blend with the lemon, the avocado and jojoba oils, and the egg yolks, into a smooth paste. Apply to skin. Leave on for 20 minutes and rinse with lemon water. Prepare lemon water from the juice of 2 lemons to 1 quart (1 l) warm water.

For cleansing and freshening

LEMON–MILK CLEANSING SOLUTION

Ingredients: 1 lemon, 3½ oz. (100 ml) milk, 1 tbsp. (15 ml) honey

Application: Squeeze out the lemon juice. Mix into milk and add honey. Saturate a cotton ball with this mixture and gently dab your skin with it. Leave on for 3 to 5 minutes. Then rinse your face as usual with plenty of clear, warm water.

LEMON WATER FOR WRINKLES

Ingredients: 2 lemons, 1 shot glass warm water

Application: Small wrinkles disappear when exposed on a regular basis to the astringent properties of lemon juice. Squeeze juice from the lemons and pour into the water. Stir well. Dab daily, morning and night, onto wrinkles with a soft pad.

LEMON–COGNAC SOLUTION FOR PIMPLES AND BLACKHEADS

Ingredients: 1 lemon, 1 tsp. (5 ml) cognac

Application: Squeeze lemon juice and blend with cognac. Saturate a Q-Tip with the solution and dab several times a day onto pimples and blackheads.

LEMON–HONEY WATER FOR ROUGH SKIN

Ingredients: 1 tbsp. (15 ml) honey, 1 cup (250 ml) water, 1 lemon
Application: Mix honey into water. Squeeze the juice of the lemon and add. Saturate a cotton ball with this solution and apply to areas of rough skin, or, in the case of hands, soak the afflicted area in the solution.

For Your Hair

Use the power of lemons to take care of your hair. The ingredients in lemons promote a healthy scalp and give your hair a silky sheen.

LEMON SHAMPOO FOR GREASY HAIR

Ingredients: 5 tsp. (25 ml) soapbark, 2 cups (500 ml) water, 1 lemon, 2 egg yolks, 5 drops lemon oil
Application: Add the soapbark to the water and gradually bring to a boil, letting it steep afterwards for 10 minutes. Allow to cool to body temperature. In the meantime you can squeeze the lemon juice. Mix the egg yolks, the lemon juice and the lemon oil into the cooled mixture. Wash your hair with this shampoo. It not only regulates the oil level of the scalp, but it will give your hair a pleasant lemon scent.

LEMON CONDITIONER FOR DULL HAIR

Ingredients: 1 lemon, 2 cups (500 ml) water, 2 tbsp. (30 ml) olive oil

The power of lemons against freckles: unwanted freckles disappear if they are treated regularly over an extended period of time with lemon juice.

Rinse your hair with the juice of half a lemon diluted with 1 cup (250 ml) lukewarm water and your hair will be shiny. The solution neutralizes the last traces of shampoo if you rinse with it after washing your hair. There is no need to wash out the rinse.

Application: Squeeze out lemon juice and add to water, followed by olive oil. Heat to body temperature and massage into hair. Wrap hair in towel. Leave conditioning treatment in hair for 30 to 45 minutes. Then rinse thoroughly with clear water.

Baths

Baths with lemon juice are beneficial to both body and soul: the scent of the essential oils in the steam rising from the bathwater acts as aromatherapy on the emotional and psychological level,

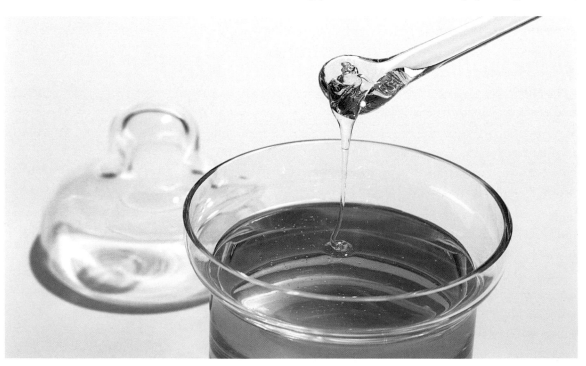

while the lemon substances in the bath regenerate your skin. Let yourself be spoiled—with lemon baths from nature's garden!

Skin-conditioning lemon–whey bath

Ingredients: 5 lemons, 8 drops lemon oil, 2 quarts (2 l) whey
Application: Squeeze the juice out of the lemons and stir into whey together with lemon oil. Pour into a full bathtub with a water temperature of 93 to 97 degrees Fahrenheit (34–36°C). Soak in the tub for 15 to 30 minutes, enjoying the scent and the feel of the gentle essences on your skin.

Morning lemon bath for stimulation

Ingredients: 1 lemon, water, 1 tbsp. (15 ml) honey, 5 drops lemon oil, 2 drops each of rosemary and eucalyptus oil
Application: Slice the lemon the evening before you take this bath and place in a bowl. Cover with water and let draw overnight. In the morning, pour this water and the lemon slices, together with the honey blended with the lemon, rosemary and eucalyptus oils, into a full bathtub. Soak for 15 minutes. You'll feel totally restored and have a fresh start to your day.

Lemon cure for tired feet

Ingredients: 1 lemon, 5 drops lemon oil, 5 drops lavender oil, 1 tbsp. (15 ml) cream
Application: Squeeze the juice out of the lemon before taking your footbath. Blend the remaining ingredients and add to a small tub of warm water. Soak feet for 15 minutes. Massage lemon juice into feet immediately after bath.

Whey contains all the valuable elements of milk in concentrated form. It has long been known as a beautifier of the skin. If you cannot get it at your grocer, you can replace it in your bath with buttermilk.

CHAPTER 6

Lemon Recipes

for the Kitchen

You can break dried
lemon peel into small
pieces and add it to
whole peppercorns in the
grinder. You can grind the
lemon pepper right onto
the food and so avoid the
tiresome grating.

Modern cuisine is unimaginable without lemons. We have gathered a number of special recipes for you in which the unique ingredients of the lemon combine ideally with the other ingredients, in terms of both health benefits and taste. A slightly different approach to enjoyment and doing something good for your health at the same time!

Sweetening and Flavoring with Lemon Aroma

LEMON SUGAR

Ingredients: dried peel of 3 lemons, 7½ oz. (200 g) sugar

Preparation: Use a small rasp to remove the lemon peel, grind to a fine powder and mix into sugar. The lemon peel should be well dried; otherwise the sugar will become lumpy.

Lemon sugar, enriched with the valuable pectin in the peel, is ideal for sweetening fruit salads or other fruit preparations, desserts, muesli or tea.

LEMON PEPPER

Ingredients: dried peel of 2 small lemons, 1¾ oz. (50 g) black pepper
Preparation: Grind the lemon peel into a fine powder with a small rasp, and mix into pepper. The lemon peel must be absolutely dry; otherwise the pepper will become lumpy. Lemon pepper is ideal for adding flavor to many meals usually prepared with black pepper, to which the slight aroma of citrus is now added.

LEMON OIL

Ingredients: 3 lemons, 3 cups (750 ml) olive oil, 8 cloves garlic
Preparation: Peel the lemons. Take care to peel in thin strips, leaving the bitter inner peel on the lemon. Place in skillet and cover abundantly with olive oil. Heat, and let the peel steep for 5 minutes. Take skillet off heat and let cool.

In the meantime, you can peel the garlic cloves and crush them. Pour the remaining olive oil into a canning jar. Add the oil from the skillet together with the lemon peel and the crushed garlic. Let the oil stand for 2 weeks and it is ready to use.

Once opened, it should be stored in the fridge. Lemon oil is ideally suited for adding a gentle touch of citrus flavor to many delicious salads, for frying and as a base for marinades.
Tip: If you use safflower oil instead of olive oil and omit the garlic, you can also use lemon oil for baking cookies or cakes.

LEMON VINEGAR

Ingredients: 4 lemons, 3 cups (750 ml) apple vinegar
Preparation: Peel lemons by hand, taking care not to include the

When cooking and baking, honey can be substituted for sugar. Simply divide the quantity of sugar in half to give you the proper amount (1 cup sugar = 1/2 cup honey). In certain recipes (such as salad dressings, sauces and drinks) an equal quantity of honey should be used (1 tsp. = 1 tsp.).

Olive oil stored in the refrigerator tends to become cloudy. Don't worry: the oil retains its quality and will regain its normal appearance at room temperature.

Lemon vinegar—vinegar to which lemon juice has been added—is available in most stores. But you can make it yourself using apple vinegar. That way you benefit from the combined salutary qualities of apple vinegar and lemons.

bitter white layer underneath the top layer of skin. Squeeze out the juice and pour into a 1 quart (1 l) canning jar together with lemon peel. Heat apple vinegar to 120 to 140 degrees Fahrenheit (50–60ºC) and pour onto the peel and lemon juice in the jar.

Seal tightly and shake well. Store for 2 weeks at room temperature. During this ripening time you should give the mixture a vigorous shake every second day. After 2 weeks you can pour the lemon vinegar through a fine sieve. Lemon vinegar is excellent for dressing fresh salad and as a basis for marinades, for example for meat.

Nutrition facts: This lemon vinegar also contains the vitamins, minerals and trace elements present in apple vinegar. These include several vitamins from the B group, vitamin E, vitamin A, beta carotene, calcium, calium, sodium, magnesium, phosphorus, sulphur, silicium, iron, and the fluoride that is so important for dental health.

Dressings, Spreads and Marinades

LEMON DRESSING FOR FRUIT SALAD

Ingredients: 6 lemons, 3 tbsp. (45 ml) thistle or wheat germ oil, 2 tsp. (10 ml) sugar or 2 tsp. (10 ml) honey, 1 pinch salt
Preparation: Squeeze juice out of lemons and blend well with other ingredients. This dressing is ideal for fruit salads.

LEMON–EGG SPREAD

Ingredients: 5 lemons, 5¼ oz. (150 g) butter, 2 tbsp. (30 ml) clear honey, 7 oz. (200 g) sugar, 4 eggs, 1 egg yolk
Preparation: Rasp off the lemon peel, squeeze out the juice and

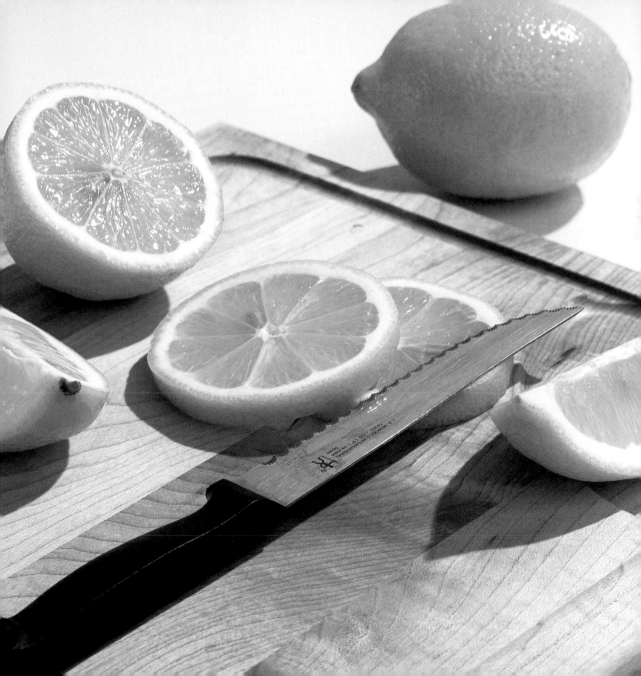

Caution: **Whenever you use lemons in your cooking, do not use pots or utensils that are made of aluminum. The acid of lemons extracts tiny traces of aluminum from the cookware, and this will give the meal a metallic taste and bleach the food colors. Use enameled or stainless steel pots.**

blend together. Warm butter over minimal heat to melt. Blend in honey and sugar until both are fully dissolved. Beat the 4 eggs until they are slightly creamy. Together with additional egg yolk and juice mixture, fold gently into butter. Allow to thicken while stirring constantly over low heat, until it reaches the consistency of jam. Let cool to room temperature and put into small jars. This is a tasty and healthy spread for bread, baguettes, toast or biscuits.

SAVORY LEMON BUTTER

Ingredients: 5¼ oz. (150 g) butter, 2 lemons, ¼ bunch finely chopped parsley, 1 pinch black pepper

Preparation: Warm butter to soften but not melt. Stir in freshly squeezed juice of the lemons, parsley and pepper. Pour butter into ice-cube container and harden in fridge. Savory lemon butter is an excellent condiment for pan-fried fish, meat and vegetable dishes, or as a spread on toast.

ASIAN LEMON MARINADE

Ingredients: 2 lemons, 2 cloves garlic, 1½ oz. (50 ml) dark soy sauce, 1 pinch powdered ginger, ⅘ cup (200 ml) sunflower or wheat germ oil, ½ cup (125 ml) dry white wine, 1 tsp. (5 ml) brown sugar or 1 tsp. (5 ml) honey

Preparation: Squeeze the juice out of both lemons. Peel garlic and crush. Add lemon juice and garlic to remaining ingredients and stir until brown sugar is dissolved. This lemon marinade is excellent for all types of meat. Marinate for at least 1½ hours.

LEMON MARINADE FOR BBQ

Ingredients: 2 lemons, 1 cup (250 ml) olive oil, 1 tbsp. (15 ml) apple vinegar, 1 tsp. (5 ml) brown sugar or 1 tsp. (5 ml) of honey, 3 cloves of garlic, 1 tsp. (5 ml) mustard (sweet or spicy according to taste), 1 pinch salt

Preparation: Squeeze juice out of lemons and add to olive oil. Stir in apple vinegar and sugar. Peel garlic, crush and add to mixture. Season to taste with mustard and salt.

This is an ideal and quick marinade for beef or chicken before grilling. It not only gives the meat a zesty flavor, but it also neutralizes any carcinogens that may be released by grilling.

Hot Drinks and Healing Teas

LEMON GRASS TEA WITH LEMON

Ingredients: 2 tsp. (10 ml) dried lemon grass, 1 cup (250 ml) water, 1 tbsp. (15 ml) freshly squeezed lemon juice, honey to taste

Preparation: Pour hot water over lemon grass. Let steep for 10 minutes, pour through sieve and add lemon juice. If you do not like the unsweetened tea, add honey to taste.

This tea is especially soothing for stomach and digestive ailments, fever, lack of appetite and nervous agitation. Drink 3 cups per day, slowly and in small sips.

BALM-MINT TEA WITH LEMON

Ingredients: 1 cup (250 ml) water, 1 heaped tbsp. (15 ml) balm-mint leaves (obtainable from your pharmacist, and in health food, tea or herbal specialty shops), 2 tbsp. (30 ml) freshly squeezed lemon juice, honey to taste.

To make a refreshing lemonade, take the zest of 1 lemon and the juice of 6, mix with 1 quart (1 l) water and add 2 oz. (50 g) sugar. Stir well and chill. Serve with ice cubes and a few fresh peppermint leaves.

Try serving this delicious dessert to your guests: lemon–egg liqueur makes a delicious sauce for a cup of ice cream with berries, whipped cream topping and wafers.

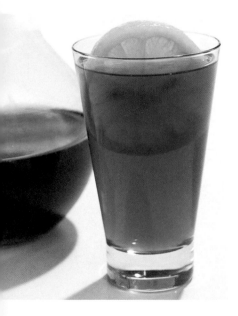

Preparation: Boil water, pour over balm-mint leaves and let steep for 10 minutes. You can then remove the leaves. Let cool to body temperature and add freshly squeezed lemon juice. Sweeten to taste with honey.

Zesty Drinks

LEMON–EGG LIQUEUR

Ingredients: 8 egg yolks, 14 oz. (400 g) sugar or 14 oz. (400 g) honey, 12 lemons, 1 vanilla pod, 2 cups (500 ml) rum (54%), about 1 cup (250 ml) milk

Preparation: Combine egg yolks and sugar in mixing bowl and beat to a froth. Squeeze lemon juice and add. Halve the vanilla pod, remove the bean and stir into mixture. Add rum and enough of the milk so that the liqueur won't be too runny.

LEMON BUTTERMILK (SERVES 4)

Ingredients: 5 egg yolks, 1¾ oz. (50 g) sugar or 1¾ oz. (50 g) honey, 2 lemons, 9 oz. (250 g) buttermilk

Preparation: Pour egg yolks into mixing bowl and stir in sugar until fully dissolved. Blend the egg–sugar mixture with the lemon juice into the buttermilk and stir well. Chill.

Now it's ready to serve—preferably on a hot summer afternoon. The milk is refreshing and healthy, a good replacement for a snack.

Index